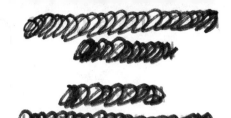

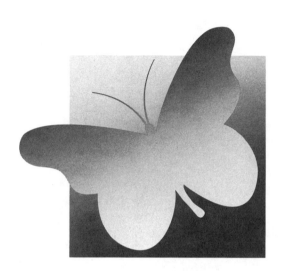

A New Beginning

Workbook I

3D

Diet, Discipline & Discipleship

10th Printing, January 1998

© Creative Joys, Inc. d/b/a 3D
P. O. Box 897
Orleans, MA 02653
ISBN #: 0-941478-70-X

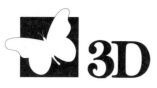

3D

Diet, Discipline & Discipleship

This workbook contains daily devotional readings, a recommended Bible reading, Bible study questions and your memory verse for each week.

The Daily Devotionals and Bible Study will be of invaluable help to you as you progress through them week by week and theme by theme. The scripture, the devotions and the questions are carefully chosen and organized in such a manner that God uses them uniquely. Many emotions, conflicts and struggles will surface, as you prayerfully read the scriptures and devotions and answer the probing questions.

The workbook devotionals are your own private tools for discovery and inspiration. Through them your entire group will be thinking and praying along the same theme each week. You will be amazed at how God uses this workbook as a catalyst to enrich the sharing in your group.

Through the 3D progam, God is starting a work in your life. Don't ever be discouraged. Take one step at a time and watch what the Lord does for you in it.

God bless you in your 3D Journey. Don't forget to let us hear from you!

The Lordship of Christ

"God has highly exalted Him . . . that at the name of Jesus every knee should bow . . . and every tongue confess that Jesus Christ is Lord, to the glory of God the Father."

Philippians 2:9-11

Jesus is Lord

Daily Reading: Acts 2:22-24, 32-42

Let all the house of Israel therefore know assuredly that God has made Him both Lord and Christ, this Jesus whom you crucified. (v. 36)

The word slips too easily from our tongues: "Lord!" But when Peter preached this sermon on the Day of Pentecost, it was no glib profession for him. The word *Kurios* had a very special meaning in that day. This was the term used for the Emperor and for the "gods" which people worshipped in that time. It meant "authority and power," and an individual was responsible to be obedient to his "lord."

Herein lies the heart of the problem for most of us as Christians. How glad we were, "when all was sin and shame," to welcome Jesus as Christ, Messiah, Anointed Saviour, who came to us in our need, bound up our wounds, and forgave and cleansed us by His own sacrificial offering on the Cross! Words can never describe what that reality means to anyone who has been convicted of sin by the Holy Spirit and has found the glorious freedom of forgiveness.

But where we have the trouble is in translating the genuine sense and knowledge of how much we owe Him for His love, into daily obedience to Him as Lord. Here we need help!

"Not everyone who says to me, Lord, Lord, shall enter the kingdom of heaven, but he who does the will of my Father who is in heaven." (Matthew 7:21)

A Prayer: *Father, forgive me that I have failed so often to do the good that I knew and have done the evil that I hate. Heal me, body, soul and spirit, that my life may show forth Your praise and glory. You have become my Saviour. By Your grace, I choose this day to make You Lord of all my life, including* _____ , _____ , and _____ . *In the Name of Jesus. Amen.*

> Behold a sinner, dearest Lord
> Encouraged by Thy gracious word
> Would venture near to seek the bread
> By which Thy children here are fed.
>
> *(Anon.)*

Ruler of All Nature

Daily Reading: Mark 4:35-41

Who is this, that even wind and sea obey Him? (v. 41)

Our Lord is a mighty God! At His command seas are quiet and winds are still. His will and His word are greater than all the forces of nature, for by His will they exist and are.

"Worthy art thou, our Lord and God, to receive glory and honor and power, for thou didst create all things, and by thy will they existed and were created." (Revelation 4:11)

It is important for me to recognize that Jesus is the Lord and Ruler of my universe. As I move about this day, I would see Him at work, and see the expression of His will and wisdom in the ordinary things as well as the big things. Not only in the stormy sea, but in the rustling grass, in the songs of birds, the passing of clouds or sunshine, I would see His creative and providential Hand.

Fairest Lord Jesus, Ruler of all nature,
O Thou of God and man the Son,
Thee would I cherish, Thee would I honor
Thou my soul's glory, joy, and crown.

Most of us make God smaller than He really is, by our limited faith. Like the people of Nazareth, whose lack of faith kept Jesus from doing many mighty works among them, we limit Him. Low vision, low aim, little faith, little results.

As I set out on this course of discipline, I would take high aim, heed the upward call, and keep my eyes on Him who is Ruler of all!

A Prayer: *We praise You, O Lord. We praise You in Your sanctuary. We praise You in Your mighty firmament! We praise You for Your mighty deeds; we praise You for Your excellent greatness! Not only with our lips, O Lord, but in our lives, by giving up ourselves to Your service. In Jesus' Name. Amen.*

1. How can you keep your vision of the Lord a large vision and still be aware of Him in the little things of your life?

2. What is the greatest and most loving thing God has done for you?

Lord of the Commonplace

Daily Reading: I Kings 20:26-30

Because the Syrians have said, "The Lord is a god of the hills but he is not a god of the valleys," therefore I will give all this great multitude into your hand, and you shall know that I am the Lord. (v. 28)

Syria made a big mistake by thinking that God was not in the valley! Apparently she respected His power on the hills, but thought she could get away with whatever she chose when it came to fighting in the valleys.

To me, the valley symbolizes the commonplace. There are no grand visions, no far horizons. Just the plodding, everyday commonplace. How easy it is to get lost in it, to forget what we saw when our hearts were lifted up on the mountaintop of inspiration. Now the vision has faded, and we are back to *reality.*

Is He the Lord of the Commonplace, or not? Here is where you must *absolutely* let the necessity of it press you to Him. For He is Lord of the Commonplace, else the whole structure falls and great is the ruin of it!

Writing about Carl Sandburg's life, Ben Hecht says, "The commonplace is the nightingale that sings in his poetry. Out of him the ordinary look of life spoke with sudden, vivid meanings, as if someone had washed the staleness from its face and uncovered its deeply human gleams."

Jesus does that with our commonplaceness, the ordinary tasks, relationships, worries, concerns and hopes that make up our lives.

In these weeks, we need to know Jesus in the common places. He is there, and He is Lord. Don't fail to seek Him!

A Prayer: *Grant us, O Lord, to pass this day in gladness and in peace, without stumbling and without stain; that, reaching the eventide victorious over all temptation, we may praise Thee, the eternal God, who art blessed, and dost govern all things, world without end. Amen.* *(Mozarabic Liturgy)*

1. What can you do to become more aware of Jesus in the ordinary tasks of your day?

2. How have you discovered Jesus' care in your commonplace activities?

Lord of the Mountains

Daily Reading: Isaiah 49:8-13

And I will make all my mountains a way. (v. 11a)

Mountains not only symbolize inspiration, such as the Mount of Transfiguration, but also that which is impossible and impassible for us. We all have our mountains of difficulties!

But stop and think! The mountain you face, which seems so hard to climb, is "His mountain." "I will make all *my* mountains a way," says the Lord. Whatever the difficult circumstance in your life at this moment, God in His great mercy and love for you has made that His circumstance. If it were yours alone, you would have reason to feel discouraged. But it is not yours alone. "For the Lord has comforted his people, and will have compassion on His afflicted."

Although you may long for greater ease, less demanding tasks, a more level road, this mountain way He calls you to walk is His way. Not only does He call you to it, but He promises to be with you.

The way may seem hard, even dreary. But look up! Keep plodding onward. The heavenly company is cheering you on, and Jesus Himself, "the Pioneer and Perfector of our faith" supplies you with secret strength against all temptations *when you abandon all for Him.*

We *need* the mountain way. No other way leads to the fulfilment and fulness of life He offers.

> I know not where the road will lead
> I follow day by day,
> Or where it ends, I only know I walk the King's highway!
> I know not if the way is long, and no one else can say;
> But rough or smooth, up hill or down, I walk the King's highway.
>
> *(Evelyn Atwater Cummins)*

A Prayer: *O God, who has commanded us to be perfect, as Thou art perfect; put into my heart, I pray Thee, a continual desire to obey Thy holy will. Teach me day by day what Thou wouldest have me to do, and give me grace and power to fulfill the same. May I never from love of ease, decline the path which Thou pointest out, nor, for fear of shame, turn away from it. Amen.*

(Henry Alford, 1810-1871)

1. When the way is smooth and easy, whose strength do we usually rely on? Why?

2. When the way gets hard, Jesus often becomes more real to us. Why?

Lord of Our Relationships

Daily Reading: Colossians 3:12-16

If any one has a complaint against another, forgiving each other as the Lord has forgiven you. (v. 13)

In the Lord's prayer we are taught to pray, "Forgive us our trespasses (or sins) as we forgive those who trespass (or sin) against us." This is the acid test of our sincerity before a holy and all-seeing God. Before Him, the secrets of all hearts are open, and we cannot hide even that which is hidden from us. Yet every time we pray in the words Jesus taught us, we ask God to forgive us *only* as we forgive others. A frightening thought!

Many of us have learned to bury and hide our negative and unforgiving feelings towards others. We know they are wrong, and so we bury them away, like a dog burying a bone in the backyard. After a while, we may even have a hard time remembering what it was. But it lies there, unresolved and unforgiven, unless from the heart, we truly forgive.

Our buried resentments, often going back to the early days of our lives, can be the unconscious and hidden source of many difficulties—including the way we feel about ourselves, the way we eat, the way we worry about how others feel about us, and on and on. Only the Spirit of Truth can unearth that which we have so carefully hidden, and bring it to light, that *real* healing and forgiveness can happen.

Ask the Spirit of Truth to bring up the hidden resentments and take them to the Cross of Jesus. There, seeing how greatly you have wronged and sinned against a loving and holy God, do not refuse to forgive those who have hurt and wronged you! You cannot truly be free unless you let Him be the Lord of your Relationships.

A Prayer: *That it may please thee to forgive our enemies, persecutors, and slanderers, and to turn their hearts: we beseech thee to hear us, good Lord . . . . That it may please thee to give us true repentance, to forgive us all our sins, negligences, and ignorances; and to endue us with the grace of thy Holy Spirit to amend our lives according to thy holy Word: we beseech thee to hear us, good Lord.*

(from the Litany, Book of Common Prayer

1. Make a list of the people who have influenced your life. Ask yourself the question, "Do I hold anything against anyone on this list?"

Lord of Our Thought Life

Daily Reading: II Corinthians 10:1-6

We destroy arguments and every proud obstacle to the knowledge of God, and take every thought captive to obey Christ. (v. 5)

Who is in control of your thought life, the secret things that fill your mind? Is Jesus Lord of your thought life?

The mind is the battleground where Satan attacks God's children. He uses every subtlety, every temptation, every imagination he can in order to lure and distract God's children away from the path of obedience and life.

He especially uses our *rightness* and *guilt.* On the one hand, the object is to keep us from confessing our wrongness that we might be cleansed and set free, and on the other, the guilt is meant to paralyze and enervate us.

If in our thoughts we harbor jealousies, envyings, resentments, and the like, we will eventually act out of those thoughts. For out of the heart are the issues of life.

"Jesus wants to be Lord of your thought life—let Him!"* Let Him begin to take control of your thoughts by bringing them to Him in confession and repentance whenever you realize that you have gotten into darkness. Don't despair, but allow Him to "take them captive" into obedience to Him.

Fenelon, counseling one who was entertaining imaginary conversations, said, "When you perceive that your imagination is beginning to work, be satisfied with turning to God, without directly combating these fancies. Let them drop, occupying yourselves in some useful way."**

Give thanks, knowing that God is working with you to bring your thoughts under the Lordship of Christ!

A Prayer: *God be in my head, and in my understanding.*
God be in my eyes, and in my looking.
God be in my mouth, and in my speaking.
God be in my heart, and in my thinking.
God be at my end, and at my departing.

(Old Sarum Primer, 1558, Salisbury, England)

1. What thoughts do you find are the most distracting for you?

---

*Cay and Judy.
**Fenelon, *The Royal Way of the Cross,* p. 49. Published by Paraclete Press, ©1982.

King of Kings and Lord of Lords

Daily Reading: Philippians 2:1-11

Therefore God has highly exalted Him and bestowed on Him the name which is above every name. (v. 9)

Let us think today about that Name. It was not always so exalted and honored! Even today, sadly, it is used in blasphemy and cursing, often taken in vain!

But it is the Name above every name. In the beginning, the Word dwelt with God and was God. The Son, who is in the bosom of the Father, knew the worship of all the heavenly host.

But though He was "in the form of God" (v. 6), He did not hold on to His divine glory and privileges, but emptied Himself and took the "form of a servant." He gave up what was His by right and became what we are, sin excepted.

In that form, lowly, unnoticed, the Carpenter of Nazareth grew up, the son of Mary. But obedience to the Father's will carried Him out into Jerusalem, and all the countryside, and after a brief ministry, they arrested Him on a false charge, beat Him almost to death, and they crucified Him between two thieves outside the walls of the city. His Name was in total shame. "He was numbered among the transgressors."

But that Name, the human name, Jesus, has been borne with total faithfulness to the Father's will. He had allowed no shame, no rejection, no pain or failure to keep Him from doing His Father's will. And that life of perfect obedience is now offered to God willingly as a sacrifice, for the salvation of all those who were lost in disobedience. Moreover, He has now set them free from their life-long bondage, and given them a new possibility, a new freedom to obey from the heart, by the power of His Spirit. He even allows them to be called by His name—*Christians*.

Having walked this same path that we walk, He is able to strengthen and help those whom He calls brethren. "For because He Himself has suffered and been tempted, He is able to help those who are tempted." (Hebrews 2:18) That means you—today.

A Prayer: *Lord Jesus Christ, Keeper and Preserver of all things, let Thy right hand guard us by day and by night, when we sit at home, and when we walk abroad, when we lie down and when we rise up, that we may be kept from all evil, and have mercy upon us sinners. Amen.* *(St Nerses of Clajes, 4th century)*

1. Jesus gave up His rights. What rights, opinons and demands do you have that keep Him from being Lord of your life?

2. As you look at your own life, where do you recognize you prefer to be served rather than be a servant? Why?

Week Review

There is a scripture in John 4 which states that "my food is to do the will of God." You are, to the best of your ability, trying to do the will of God through your commitment to the 3D program. We know you will be blessed.

1. In the Daily Devotional, which day that talked about the Lordship of Christ did you find most meaningful?

2. Where did you recognize that Jesus Christ was not the Lord of your life?

3. What one strong opinion do you have that you know God would like you to stop hanging on to?

4. Did you lose any weight this week? (Or gain it, if you are in the program to gain!)

SPIRITUAL JOURNAL

You shall be filled with all good things if you seek the Kingdom of God, which is Jesus.

M. Cay & M. Judy

Why Discipline?

"For the moment all discipline seems painful rather than pleasant; later it yields the peaceful fruit of righteousness to those who have been trained by it."

Hebrews 12:11

Week 2, Day 1

Those Who Have Been Trained by It

Daily Reading: Hebrews 12:1-11

For the moment all discipline seems painful . . . later it yields the peaceful fruit of righteousness to those who have been trained by it. (v. 11)

"To those who have been trained by it." We have a choice in anything that anyone says to us or anything that happens to us, either to let work for us, or to refuse to let it work for us.

Pressure can turn us into something hard and bitter, or it can break us and make us soft and merciful. It depends on whether or not we "have been trained by it."

A word of correction spoken by husband, wife, parent, employer, or friend—can either be a cause of anger and stored-up resentment, or we can let it work for us, and be trained by it.

The choice is *ours*. The person who would become an athlete must undergo *painful* discipline to get into shape. Ask anyone who has. The person who would become a musician must sacrifice hours and hours of practice, day after day. Sometimes it is inwardly very painful. But it must be done if the goal is to be achieved. There could be no army without discipline!

We Christians cannot afford to be soft on ourselves if we would become the praises of His glory. We cannot afford to go on undisciplined, living by the whim and feeling of the moment if we would grow in Christ. The diet and disciplines we face during these weeks are only tools to help us become better soldiers, disciples, followers of Jesus. The goal is well worth the effort. The discipline may not be pleasant at the moment, but keep your eye on the goal—and on the Leader. He has already endured His discipline!

A Prayer: *Lord, open my eyes to see how Your disciplines are being worked in my life, and give me grace to cooperate with You, so that I may be trained by them to become what You want me to be. I ask this in the Name of Jesus Christ my Lord. Amen.*

1. How can you cooperate with God so that He can turn pressure into a blessing in your life?

2. As you look at your life, are there areas where you are demanding your own way and are unwilling to face the discipline that you need in order to grow? List.

16

Let Us Rejoice in Our Sufferings

Daily Reading: Romans 5:1-11

More than that, let us rejoice in our sufferings, knowing that suffering produces endurance, and endurance produces character, and character produces hope, and hope does not disappoint us . . . . (vv. 3-5a)

Ours is not a "suffering" religion. There is not glorification of suffering for its own sake. Jesus says to His followers, "I will not leave you desolate," (John 14:18); "Peace I leave with you," (John 14:27); "These things I have spoken to you, that my joy may be in you, and that your joy may be full," (John 15:11). Joy is a keynote of His life and whenever He is present "there is fullness of joy!"

What, then, can Paul mean about rejoicing in our sufferings?

First, we can rejoice, knowing that God is *using* the suffering for our good, and it is not "going to waste"!

Second, we can rejoice in knowing the presence of Jesus in ways we cannot know when everything is bright and pleasant. Stars can be seen only at night, and many hidden things of God can we receive only in and through our suffering. As we suffer out of whatever it is which brings us pain, we know Him in a deeper and more intimate way.

"The love of Jesus, what it is
None but His loved ones know."

Finally, we can rejoice, as Jesus did, "for the joy set before him." The Cross was not an easy thing for Him. Neither is our cross an easy thing for us. But the joy set before Him—the hope that beyond the suffering there was a new reality waiting—carried Him through!

A Prayer: *O loving Jesus, help me to set aside all self-pity and false ideas about how hard my lot in life is! I look at what You suffered and am ashamed of how little I am willing to suffer and how easily I say "Enough!" Give me grace to share the joy You offer me even in the midst of my sufferings. I thank You for it, Lord Jesus. Amen.*

1. How can self-pity take away all the constructive value of suffering and turn it into a destructive experience?

2. How can you cooperate with God so that He can turn suffering into a blessing in your life?

Week 2, Day 3

Adding to Your Faith

Daily Reading: II Peter 1:1-11

If these things are yours and abound, they keep you from being ineffective or unfruitful in the knowledge of the Lord Jesus Christ. (v.8)

Salvation is a free gift! We come to the Lord in our helplessness and need, and He saves us by His own grace and through the sacrifice of His own life on the Cross! It stands forever as the great, unfathomable mystery of our faith. It is the eternal good news. Catherine Hankey's familiar gospel song says it well:
> I love to tell the story,
> 'Twill be my theme in glory
> To tell the old, old story
> Of Jesus and His love.

It remains the touchstone against which everything else must be measured. Our Hope and our Salvation is in Who He is and what He has done for us!

The Apostle here, however, gives us an important reminder that even in this knowledge of His love we may become ineffective and unfruitful—unless we do our part. Paul referred to himself and Apollos as "God's fellow workers." Peter here challenges us to "add to your faith." The list of virtues is impressive, even staggering: "Virtue, knowledge, self-control, steadfastness, godliness, brotherly affection, and love." It shows us where the inner battles are to be fought and where our work as Christian men and women truly lies—for most of us have far to go before achieving all these qualities.

Let God speak to you about where you need to pay closer attention to one or more of these areas in your life. The disciplines of 3D should prove helpful in facing them. Do not let disappointment in yourself or discouragement rob you of eventual victory!

A Prayer: *Merciful and gracious God! Let Thy grace strengthen my faith, awaken my love, and maintain my hope. Let Thy grace be my joy and glory, my comfort and life. Let Thy grace create meekness, humility, patience, devotion and prayer in me, for Thy grace works all good within me. Amen.*

(Johann Arndt, 1551-1621)

1. How can you keep from letting discouragement or disappointment in yourself rob you of eventual victory?

As a Man Disciplines His Son

Daily Reading: Deuteronomy 8:5-16

Know then in your heart, as a man disciplines his son, the Lord your God disciplines you. (v. 5)

Israel was taught to see. God's love and God's training as the great realities of her life. God had set His love on her, but she was by nature a rebellious people. Yet God did not cease to love her!

"Sons I have reared and brought up, but they have rebelled against me. The ox knows its owner, and the ass its master's crib; but Israel does not know, my people do not understand." (Isaiah 1:2b,3)

In this Deuteronomy passage, we are reminded of the forty-year wilderness experience Israel had before reaching the Promised Land. They were being led out of bondage. But the way led "through the great and terrible wilderness, with its fiery serpents and scorpions and thirsty ground where there was no water. . . ." And the reason for all this was "that he might humble and test (or prove) you, *to do you good in the end*" (vv. 15, 16). God's love and God's discipline.

Without discipline we become presumptuous, and take for granted His love and grace. With discipline, we can enter into a loving relationship as those who have learned both their own need of it and the amazing love behind it. See discipline as from One whose will is "to do you good in the end."

A Prayer: *Your steadfast love, O Lord, never ceases. Your mercies never come to an end. They are new every morning. Great is Your faithfulness. The Lord is my portion; therefore I will hope in Him. Amen.*

(Adapted from Lamentations 3:22-24)

1. How do you come to really know that God's discipline is His love?

2. Where do you see God's Fatherly discipline in your life?

Week 2, Day 5

As a Good Soldier

Daily Reading: II Timothy 2:1-11

Take your share of suffering as a good soldier of Christ Jesus. (v. 3)

Take your share. What is your share of suffering? Does it seem that you have been allotted *more* than your share? Have you ever wondered if the Christians in the Colosseum before the lions thought they were being asked to take more than their share, or those who were used to light the roads leading to Rome, human torches, under the wicked Nero? Or what the soldiers in the Battle of Hastings, or at Valley Forge or in the swamps of Vietnam felt? *Take your share!* We are in a spiritual battle, and it will not be won by those who give in to self-pity, self-indulgence, or self-justifying rationalizations.

As a good soldier of Christ Jesus, we are enlisted under the banner of the Cross. We have heard the call in our hearts, we have received the amazing love and forgiveness He offered us in our need. Now He says, "Behold, I send you. . ." and we find ourselves in a battle. Many Christians are surprised to find it so! Our daily disciplines are battles to be fought and won to train us for battles yet to be encountered. But remember Jesus Christ *risen from the dead!* He has won the victory!

> Must I be carried to the skies
> On flowery beds of ease,
> While others fought to win the prize
> And sailed through bloody seas!
>
> No! I must fight if I would reign!
> Increase my courage, Lord.
> I'll bear the cross, endure the pain,
> Supported by Thy Word.

A Prayer: Lord Jesus Christ: You are the Saviour and Captain of my soul. I am Yours, and I desire to be Yours this day and always. Take from me all that hinders my service to You, and give me grace to be a loyal and faithful soldier to my life's end. In Your holy Name. Amen.

1. What spiritual battles have you fought this week?

2. What hindrances do you see in your life that keep you from victory?

Ready, Aim, Fire!

Daily Reading: I Timothy 6:11-16

Fight the good fight of faith; take hold of the eternal life to which you were called when you made the good confession in the presence of many witnesses. (v. 12)

In this passage, young Timothy was urged to "aim at righteousness, godliness, faith, love, steadfastness and gentleness" (v. 11). He would not always hit the target, but he was to keep on aiming! There is no place for discouragement and no *reason* for it in the Christian life. If we get discouraged, it is because we have put too much faith in *ourselves* and too little in Jesus. It is because we have underestimated the seriousness of our condition and how radical a change following Jesus truly requires. It is because we would rather give in than fight against ourselves.

So away with discouragement! *Eternal life,* life in all its fullness and contentment is *ours* by the gift of God's grace in Jesus Christ. But we must constantly "lay hold" or "take hold" of that life, and that process means fighting the good fight against "the world, the flesh and the devil."

One of the devil's chief weapons is discouragement, and we overcome by keeping alive our remembrance of who we are and who Jesus is. We are rescued and He is the Savior! So, take aim!

> Fight the good fight with all thy might,
> Christ is thy strength and Christ thy right;
> Lay hold on life, and it shall be
> Thy joy and crown eternally.
>
> Cast care aside, lean on thy Guide;
> His boundless mercy will provide;
> Trust, and thy trusting soul shall prove
> Christ is its life and Christ its love.
>
> *(J. S. B. Monsell, 1863)*

A Prayer: In Your strength I will fight. By Your grace I shall stand. In Your Name I will win. Hallelujah! Amen.

1. Are there areas in your life you'd rather give in to than fight yourself? What are they?

2. If you've been discouraged about anything this week, how did you handle it?

Discipline and Preparedness

Daily Reading: Matthew 25:1-13

But the wise took flasks of oil with their lamps. (v. 4)

What has discipline to do with preparedness? Today's scripture ties them together, because to be disciplined is to be in a state of readiness. As we fight against self-love, self-indulgence, and carelessness, we are "tuned-up" for whatever comes. If our prayer life, our reading of God's Word, our personal habits or our obligations are slovenly, we are like soldiers who are not prepared for the call to battle. The enemy may find us unaware!

The Lord, too, bids us be ready for His appearing. Not only at the Second Coming, or at the hour of death, but wherever He appears in our lives. Are we in a state of readiness for Him? Are we prepared to hear His Word of truth, to see His hand, to minister to "one of these little ones" in His name? All this has to do with discipline, to prepare us for whatever He has for us to do. Usually, it will be nothing great or spectacular. It may not even be religious or spiritual in the narrower sense. But if it is done "as unto the Lord," it will not lose its reward.

Let us be with the wise, who "took flasks of oil with their lamps," and be ready.

A Prayer When Tempted

Jesus, you know the temptations I feel.
You are acquainted with all my way.
You know my heart, my thoughts, my wants and desires.
O Jesus, whose will was one with the Father's, by your grace, make my will one with yours.
I offer it to you now, Lord. Have mercy on me and come to my assistance!
I claim the Name of Jesus as shield against the onslaught of Satan!
I claim the Name of Jesus as the sign of victory over these thoughts that beset me.
Jesus is Victor! Hallelujah!

1. Are there personal habits or obligations in your life that are slovenly? What are they?

2. What can you do to begin to change?

Week Review

This week the emphasis was on discipline. It has been amazing to all of us in 3D to realize how many of us see discipline as a negative thing. We cannot understand how it could be a freeing tool of God—and yet we find exactly that. The more disciplined we are, the freer we feel. It certainly is a paradox.

1. What disciplines in 3D have you found the easiest to follow?

2. What disciplines have you found the hardest?

3. What specific discipline do you want to work harder on this week?

SPIRITUAL JOURNAL

Any situation that you think you cannot possibly endure can become the very means of giving you the greatest freedom, if you allow it to.

M. Cay & M. Judy

God's Will or My Will?

"Nevertheless not my will but thine be done."

Luke 22:42

"I Seek Not My Own Will"

Daily Reading: John 5:30-44

I seek not my own will, but the will of Him who sent me. (v. 30b)

Long before Jesus was born, the Psalmist prophetically spoke of Him by the Spirit, saying, "Lo, I come; in the roll of the book it is written of me: I delight to do thy will, O my God; thy law is within my heart." (Psalm 40:7,8) Of Him it could be said, and of no other, "His will was one with the Father's will."

But this does not mean Jesus was never tempted. Even though His human nature was sinless, He nevertheless was fully human, and therefore subject to the same temptation that Adam and Eve experienced. They succumbed to the lies and seductions of Satan, but Jesus, when tempted, confronted Satan with the truth, and kept His will in complete oneness with the Father.

> O wisest love! That flesh and blood
> Which did in Adam fail
> Should strive afresh against the foe—
> Should strive and should prevail!
>
> *(John Henry Newman)*

Jesus has been tempted, and has prevailed. He knows what it means to face temptation, and *therefore* can help us when we flee to Him. He it is who can help us, and He will help us if we, like Him, will say, "I seek not my own will. Not my will, but thine be done!"

A Prayer: *Lord, our wills are not yet one with yours. We struggle to keep them for our own. Yet we have heard your call, and we have seen the fruit of yielding up our way. Take my will and make it thine, this very day. In Jesus' Name. Amen.*

1. There is a wise saying which goes like this: "I can't stop the birds from flying over my head but I can stop them from nesting in my hair." How can this be applied to the experience of temptation?

2. Why is it wise to "nip temptation in the bud"?

Teach Me To Do Thy Will

Daily Reading: Psalm 143

The Psalmist wrote in a situation of deep trouble. Such phrases as "crushed to the ground," "my spirit faints within me," and "he has made me sit in darkness," give some indication of the seriousness of his plight. In a situation like that, it would be very tempting to wallow in self-pity and to think dark, vindictive thoughts against "the enemy." In fact, some of the Psalms are very free in expressing that kind of emotional release, and we all need it at times. God seems to be saying, through the Psalms, that it is all right to recognize and express these feelings to God! After all, He knows they are there even better than we know ourselves.

But here in this Psalm, there is something more. "I have fled to thee for refuge!" (verse 9) The place to go in our struggles against the enemy is to the place of refuge. But it is not just a passive, peaceful place, where we will be patted on the head and told that everything will be all right. The very next verse says it: "Teach me to do thy will, for thou art my God!" To remain in the place of refuge, and to know the peace we all long to have inwardly, we must seek to know and to do the will of God.

"My thoughts are not your thoughts, neither are your ways my ways, says the Lord." (Isaiah 55:8) Because this is so, we need to be taught His ways and His will.

He teaches us His will in many ways, and even though we may not find His disciplines easy, there is a tremendous fulfillment in following them. We are learning as we follow. Our prayer is being answered even as we pray.

A Prayer: *Father, teach us to come to you by the One and Living Way, Jesus Christ. Keep us humble and gentle, self-denying, firm and patient, active, wise to know Your will and to discern the truth; loving, that we may learn to resemble You and our Savior, Jesus Christ, in whose name we pray. Amen.* *(Adapted)*

1. We learned today that we need to be taught His will and His ways. How are we taught His will and His ways?

2. David in the Psalms is very free in expressing his feelings. Why is this good?

Week 3, Day 3

Say or Doing?

Daily Reading: Matthew 21:23-46

Which of the two did the will of his father? (v. 31a)

Jesus told the story of the two sons who were told to go and work in their father's vineyard. The first said, "I will not," but changed his mind afterward, and went. The second answered, "I go, sir," but did not go. And then Jesus poses the question: "Which of the two did the will of his father?"

Profession is easy. The promises we make with our lips are not costly, unless we are prepared to follow through. Sometimes there comes up within us such a force of resistance and rebellion, that the first word out of our hearts is "No! I will not!" But then, by the grace of God, we begin to look at the foolish and hurtful thing we have done. We begin to repent of that within us which so resists doing God's will. We may pray. There may even be tears of repentance. But the most important thing is, we begin to see how wrong we are! And, like the first son, we repent and do what God has required of us. We may not like it. We may not enjoy doing it. But we do it anyway!

On the other hand, the most dangerous spiritual condition is the self-deception that lurks in this story. Because the second son was pleasant, because he did not outwardly oppose his father, he may even have counted himself to be a good and obedient son. Certainly most of us have done something similar, and it may take us some time to come to the realization that we are not obedient just because we think of ourselves as good Christians. We may generously overlook our own faults, but Jesus is saying here that more than lip service, more than promises, more than "Yes, I go," are required. Sooner or later, we must do the will of the Father. Better sooner than later. Better now than tomorrow. Better deeds than words.

A Prayer: *Give us such an awareness of your mercies, that with truly thankful hearts we may show forth your praise, not only with our lips, but in our lives, by giving up ourselves to your service, and by walking before you in holiness and righteousness all our days; through Jesus Christ our Lord. Amen.*

(Adapted from Morning Prayer service, Book of Common Prayer, 1979)

1. Which son are you like?

2. What does repentance mean to you?

28

Not Everyone Who Says, Lord, Lord

Daily Reading: Matthew 7:15-28

Not every one who says to me, Lord, Lord, shall enter the kingdom of heaven, but he who does the will of my Father who is in heaven. (v. 21)

As Christians, we live between what we have been and what we are to become. Our lives are in process of changing. It may seem as though we are never going to change in this or that area, but in point of fact, we are changing; we are becoming.

What are we becoming! That depends on the direction and aim of our hearts. If they are "toward the Lord," then the changes, however slow and painful, are moving towards becoming conformed to the will of God. If our hearts are set on doing our own will, following our own course, then we are changing in a negative way. Look at older people, and you can see that they show in clearer, less hidden ways what they have been becoming for many decades. It can be encouraging, and it can serve as a warning!

In another place we are told that it is not God's will that any should perish, but that all should come to eternal life. His will is life-abundant life, for all. Therefore to begin doing the will of God is not to fulfill some hard, rigid task. "For my yoke is easy, and my burden is light," Jesus said (Matthew 11:30). God's will is fulfilled as we leave our own ways, recognize our own inadequacy and sin, and begin to walk in His ways. It is not some new legalism, where all we do is to follow the new rules. It is walking by the Spirit, being guided both by inward impulse and by outward circumstances, with the help and fellowship of others, along a path of life. It is a path of LIFE, a movement from where we have been to where we are going. At times we are discouraged; at other times, we are exalted and full of joy. But we keep on moving, seeking more and more to "do the will of our Father in heaven."

Let this truth penetrate your thoughts and flood you with new zeal and hope!

A Prayer: *Thy kingdom come — in me today, O Lord. Thy will be done — in me today, O Lord, as it is by those who are perfected in the Heavenly Kingdom. For thine is the kingdom I seek. Thine is the power to accomplish it. Thine is the glory, for ever and ever. Amen.*

1. Where have you found that the will of God is not hard and rigid?

2. What specifically is God's will for you today?

If Any Man's Will Is to Do His Will . . .

Daily Reading: John 7:14-31

If any man's will is to do His will, he shall know whether this teaching is from God or whether I am speaking on my own authority. (v. 17)

With all the different doctrines, ideas and teachings that one can hear or read, it is no wonder that people feel confused. Maybe you are one who has felt this confusion, and have asked yourself the question, "How can I know? How can I be sure?" Jesus here is saying that there is a definite connection between our willingness to do God's will and our ability to know truth from falsehood. Unless there is in us a deep, underlying desire to find and do the will of God, we can be tossed about by all kinds of half-truths, quarter-truths, or down-right falsehoods. Look at the evidence all around us.

This does not mean that we always *like* doing the will of God, or that we always succeed in carrying out His will. Paul is a good example of this, when, as we know, he gave up everything to follow Christ, suffered many things—beaten, stoned, shipwrecked, rejected—and yet, writing from prison, he says, "Not that I have already obtained this (his goal), or am already perfect, but I press on to make it my own . . ." (Philippians 3:12a). His *will* was set to go on with Jesus. That is basic to everything. If we would know Him and His power in our lives, we must set our wills, like a ship set on course, or a rocket pointed for the moon— *to do his will.* In that condition, He promises that we will *know.*

When that is not our heart's desire, when there is a mixture of wanting His will and wanting our own, we can be confused. We may waver about which course to take. But when we put down our own will and choose His, in spite of all the fightings that may go on within us, then we are on the way! We do not have to stay locked in uncertainty, if we will but set our wills, over and over again, *to do his will.*

A Prayer: *Heavenly Father, send your Holy Spirit into our hearts, to direct and rule us, according to your will, to comfort us in all our afflictions, to defend us from all error, and to lead us into all truth, through Jesus Christ our Lord. Amen.*

(Book of Common Prayer, 1979)

Today's teaching talks about setting our wills to do the Will of God.
1. Why is doing God's will not always easy?

2. Give an example from your own life to illustrate your answer.

When the Will Is Defective

Daily Reading: Romans 7:13-25

I can will what is right, but I cannot do it. (v. 18b)

Has that ever been your experience? It has been mine over and over again. What it shows us is that there is much about us that we do not understand. We act out of hidden, unrecognized motivations that lie deeply buried within us. It has been the sobering experience of Christians in all ages that we can desire, but that we cannot always accomplish what is right. We need help! It seems as though we should be able to summon strength to do the will of God perfectly, but in actual experience, there is still too much of the old carnal (fleshy) nature alive in us. We are not yet sanctified and mature in Christ. So there are times when we are under the rulership of Jesus and there are times when we give expression to the old nature. One commentator says, "There is no believer, however advanced in holiness, who cannot adopt the language used here by the apostle . . . . Everyone feels that he cannot do the things he would, yet is sensible that he is guilty for not doing them. Let any man test his power by the requirement to love God perfectly at all times. Alas! How entire our inability! Yet how deep our self-loathing and self-condemnation !" *

Confronted with the defectiveness of our wills, we turn for help, not only in prayer to the Lord, but to others. By exposing our need, by giving others permission to speak truth to us, by willingness to listen to the Word of God through our sisters and our brothers in Christ, we can realize His help in a greater way. He helps us, not only through the inward grace He gives, but through the ministry of others in the Body of Christ, making us members of a Body instead of soloists in the spiritual battle. Thanks be to God for His merciful provision!

A Prayer: *O God, I thank you for my fellow members in Christ's Body, who are willing to help me in my battle against the habits and the bondage of my old carnal nature. Amen.*

Today's lesson talks of exposing our need.
1. To whom could you expose your need?

2. Why is it hard for us to expose our need?

*Jamison, Fausett and Brown, Commentary.

Living by the Will of God

Daily Reading: I Peter 4:1-19

Arm yourselves . . . so as to live for the rest of the time in the flesh no longer by human passions, but by the will of God (v. 1b, 2). Therefore let those who suffer according to God's will do right and entrust their souls to a faithful creator (v. 19).

I heard a preacher say once that when he was a child, the only time he heard about "the will of God" was when someone died. People would stand around and say in a hushed voice, "It was God's will." So, said he, when he became a man, and someone happened to mention "the will of God," he would think, "Has it come to *that?*"

How many of us, when we struggle with our own wills against His will, actually think that God's will is wrong, unkind, hard, or unfair! The one-talent man in Jesus' parable said to his master, "Master, I knew you to be a hard man, reaping where you did not sow, and gathering where you did not winnow; so I was afraid . . . ." Too often, when we want what He does not will, we hurl the same kind of accusations at God—consciously or unconsciously. And then we struggle to make His will conform to ours.

If we insist too long and too hard, God may give us up to our own wills. He often does that. But He is not obligated to make things turn out the way we thought they would or hoped they would. If we insist on our own way, we have to live with the consequences.

Living by the will of God may be a real struggle—it is for most of us. But He promises that in His will we will be cared for and blessed. We may not have all the details just the way we want them, but we will find that our wants and His will can more and more become one. Did living by our feelings (our passions) bring us freedom and peace? Why not then choose to live by His will?

A Prayer: *O Almighty and most merciful God, of thy bountiful goodness keep us, we beseech thee, from all things that may hurt us; that we, being ready both in body and soul, may cheerfully accomplish those things which thou commandest; through Jesus Christ our Lord. Amen.* *(Book of Common Prayer)*

1. Where have you seen that living by the Will of God may be a real struggle but in the long run it always brings blessings?

2. Where have you seen that insisting on having your own way leads to disaster or disappointment?

Week Review

1. Do you feel you know how to find the will of God in little things

easily _____ occasionally _____ with difficulty _____ ?

Do you feel you know how to find the will of God in big things

easily _____ occasionally _____ with difficulty _____ ?

2. Has this week's study helped you in this regard? If so, how?

3. Are you willing today to recommit yourself to go on?

SPIRITUAL JOURNAL

When you're in the will of God you have the grace for what you cannot do.
M. Cay & M. Judy

Learning to Listen

"But he who listens to me will dwell secure and will
be at ease, without dread of evil."

Proverbs 1:33

God Speaks in Many Ways

Daily Reading: Hebrews 1

In many and various ways God spoke of old to our fathers by the prophets (v. 1).

We believe in a God who speaks! *"He is There and He is Not Silent"* is the title of a book which has had wide popularity in Christian circles. This means that we have fellowship with Him, not only in what we say to Him, but in listening to what He has to say to us.

In this week's devotions and Bible study, we are thinking about the various ways God speaks. It is an important lesson for every earnest Christian to learn. Otherwise, we may end up trying to live our lives like deaf runners, who have only the distant goal in mind, but no fellowship or instruction along the way. He has not left us so bereft!

From the beginning of the Bible, God has spoken to man. First, He gave Adam and Eve instructions as to how they were to live and enjoy life on this earth. Then after they had sinned and were hiding in fear, "they heard the sound of the Lord God walking in the garden" (Gen. 3:8) and heard the voice of God calling to them. But the fruit of man's sin was banishment from that close fellowship with God, and man had to learn to listen to God's Word through men like Moses, Elijah, and other prophets.

It was a sad day in Israel when there was no one to hear from God. In I Samuel 3:1, we read, "And the word of the Lord was rare in those days; there was no frequent vision."

We know that God "is there and He is not silent." The challenge is to become sensitive to His voice. It will not always come clothed as we expect it. It will often surprise us and may even cause us pain and dismay. But His voice, His Word is life and hope.

He speaks, and list'ning to his voice	Hear him, ye deaf; his praise, ye dumb,
New life the dead receive,	Your loosened tongues employ;
The mournful broken hearts rejoice,	Ye blind, behold your Saviour come,
The humble poor believe.	And leap, ye lame, for joy!

(Charles Wesley, 1740)

A Prayer: *Make my ears attentive, O Lord, to Your voice. May I yearn to hear Your Word and be quick to perform it. For Jesus' sake. Amen.*

1. How can you become more sensitive to God's voice?

2. During these past four weeks, have you discovered God speaking to you in new ways? List. Discuss the new ways in which you've heard from God.

Listening to God's Prophet

Daily Reading: Exodus 20

You speak to us and we will hear; but let not God speak to us, lest we die. (v. 19)

In the previous chapter, Israel said to Moses, "All that the Lord has spoken we will do." God, in order to confirm to the people that He indeed was speaking by Moses, allowed them to hear the thunder of His mighty voice. The experience was so frightening that they wanted an easier way to hear from Him. From that time on, God raised up prophets to speak to the people and to their rulers.

It was an awesome responsibility to be a prophet. The prophet was accountable to God for what he said, no matter how difficult his message. Naturally, some prophets found such a task too difficult, so they would change the message or make up one of their own which was more agreeable to the hearers. One of the marks of the true prophet was that he often warned the people about where they were wrong and what would happen if they did not change. The false prophet was frequently more pleasant!

The gift of prophecy did not stop with the coming of Jesus. Indeed, the Book of Acts says that the latter day will see "your sons and daughters" prophesying. That means that there will be many who speak the divine message to His people by the power of the Holy Spirit.

When we hear someone with a word from the Lord, whether in sermon, teaching, or otherwise, are we attentive to it? Do we, like Israel, say, "All that the Lord has spoken we will do"? Or do we think to ourselves, "Who is this person to be speaking for God?" There are still false prophets, of course, and we are told "Do not despise prophesying, but test everything and hold fast what is good" (I Thess. 5:20,21). They must exalt Jesus Christ and be faithful to the written Word of God; otherwise they are not true prophets at all. But we should be humble enough to hear God through His servants whom He has called and anointed for that purpose. They have been given to the Church to build us up in the faith and to bring us to maturity in Christ.

A Prayer: *Father, give me the humility to hear Your voice through Your servants whom You have sent and ordained for this holy purpose. As they preach, teach, and speak the Word of God to me, give me ears to hear and a heart to understand. Amen.*

1. Do you find it difficult to believe that God speaks to you through other people? Why?

The Still Small Voice

Daily Reading: I Kings 19:1-18

And after the fire, a still small voice (v. 12).

Elijah had had a tremendous spiritual victory over all the prophets of Baal at Mount Carmel. The false prophets had tried in vain to prove the power of their god, and Elijah had waited, taunting them in their failure. Then, at the time of the evening sacrifice, he "repaired the altar of the Lord," which had fallen into disuse. The sacrifice was then prepared, and God answered his prayer by fire from heaven, consuming the entire sacrifice, and the altar as well! The people were impressed, to say the least! "The Lord, he is God!" they cried over and over again. And in that moment, Elijah acted—having the 450 false prophets seized and slain on the spot, seeking to rid the country and the people of the false religion which was destroying them.

Then Jezebel, the wicked queen, sent Elijah word, promising to do to him just what he had done to her Baal prophets, and Elijah was frightened. He felt alone, knowing her power over her husband the king. So he fled from the capital city and finally came to a cave many miles away, broken, full of self-pity and anger. God displayed His might in wind, earthquake, and fire—reminding Elijah that His hand is not shortened that it cannot save! But the real message came after the display, in "a still small voice."

We tend to look for God in the big things, the great and impressive displays of His miracles and His might. How easy it is to ignore the still, small voice within. He often speaks in our conscience, a little warning, a little, quiet reminder of what He wants us to do. But unless we are attentive, we will hasten on, looking for the big event. In the small things of everyday, He is still speaking.

A Prayer: *Lord, You have made us for fellowship with You. Give me ears to hear the still, small voice within. May I treasure that inward communion above all earthly delights, and grieve not Your Holy Spirit. Amen.*

1. When in your life recently have you, like Elijah, forgotten all God has done and instead you've fled into self-pity and anger?

2. How do you believe you can become more keenly aware of the "still small voice" of God speaking to you daily?

Listening to Jesus

Daily Reading: Mark 9:1-29

This is my beloved Son; listen to Him (v. 7).

How they were to listen to Jesus was very clear. They were with Him physically, and He spent much time talking to them and training them for what was to come. Even so, they did not understand much of what He was saying until after He was crucified. We may envy them and suppose it was easier. But they did not have the advantages we have. We have not only their later witnesses of His glorious resurrection and ascension to God's right hand, but we have the testimonies of twenty centuries of followers who have found Him a Friend indeed. So we need not envy the fact that listening to Him was a clear and direct thing.

Instead, we need to listen to Him today. "He speaks to me everywhere," says the songwriter. Look about you today and listen for His voice. He is the Creator of all, and not only the birds, the stars, the sun and moon "proclaim His praise," but to the listening ear come intimations, thoughts, a sense of knowing—which we can learn to identify as His voice to us, not in some vague, romantic way, not in some super-spiritual way, but as the living communication of our Living Christ.

His Words in Scripture, especially Jesus' words in the Gospels, are powerful words to us. Inwardly digest them, savor them as you read. They burned their way into the hearts of their hearers and later were "written down for our instruction" (I Corinthians 10:11). Let them burn their way into your mind as a strong word of help and guidance. He speaks through them as well as through His living Spirit today. "He that has ears to hear, let him hear."

A Prayer: *Lord Jesus, sanctify me in the truth. Thy Word is truth. Amen.*

1. Where have you had a "sense of knowing" that God is speaking to you this week?

2. When and where is it easiest for you to hear God? Why?

Listening to Scripture

Daily Reading: II Timothy 3

All Scripture is inspired by God, and profitable for teaching, for reproof, for correction, and for training in righteousness, that the man of God may be complete, equipped for every good work (vv. 16,17).

How important it is to hear God in the Holy Scriptures. It is our safeguard against untold errors, and in them is contained all things necessary for our salvation. Paul here is giving some very basic advice to his son in the faith, young Timothy. Timothy is called on to lead people who have not had the advantage he, Timothy, had in associating closely with Paul. They need someone who has learned the faith and learned it well. Paul reminds Timothy that he had been acquainted with the Scriptures since his childhood, and in another place, speaks of Timothy's mother and grandmother as having been believers before him. Now that Timothy is "on his own," so to speak, the Scriptures are a safeguard against the deceptions and deceivers he is meeting in the world.

The same is true for us today. Many erroneous and strange teachings are for sale today in the Christian marketplace. Some of them sound very attractive, and offer us quick gratification, telling us that we are wonderful and that we have nothing to worry about. Others play on guilt, fear, uncertainty about the future, and enslave their hearers in new bondages. What is the remedy against such error? The Holy Scriptures.

It is not by accident that the Church has referred to the Bible as The Word of God. It is a treasure and storehouse of divine wisdom and truth. We have been given the Holy Spirit as our enlightener and guide, and the Church itself as a check against any possible private interpretations that might lead us astray. With those two safeguards, we can open the Scriptures expectantly. They are profitable for teaching, reproof, correction, and training in righteousness. God speaks through them to our conditions. Those whom He has anointed often interpret them to our good. "Thy Word is a lamp to my feet, and a light to my path. I have laid up thy Word in my heart, that I might not sin against thee" (Psalm 119:105 and 11).

A Prayer: *O that we, discerning Its most holy learning,*
Lord, may love and fear thee, Evermore be near thee!

(Henry W. Baker, 1861)

1. Where have you allowed the Holy Spirit to speak to you specifically this week through the Scriptures themselves?

2. Do you need help to hear God speak to you through the Bible? (If your answer is yes, perhaps you could talk about this in the group, with your leaders.)

God Speaks Through Our Circumstances

Daily Reading: Isaiah 30:8-33

And though the Lord give you the bread of adversity and the water of affliction, yet your Teacher will not hide himself anymore, but your eyes shall see your Teacher, and your ears shall hear a word behind you, saying, This is the way, walk in it, when you turn to the right or when you turn to the left (vv. 20,21).

God was speaking to His people through the circumstances of their life. "Woe to the rebellious children who carry out a plan but not mine" is the first word of warning. If we insist on doing things our own way, working out our own wills, God warns us lovingly that we will come to regret it!

Israel would go through times of great affliction. She would be battered and tossed about as the great nations around her played with her like a pawn on a chessboard. But God was keeping watch. His business with Israel was to bring her, chastened and fashioned into a new time. "The Lord waits to be gracious to you" (v. 18).

It is so with us. Our ways end up in affliction, confusion and distress. Most of us know from firsthand experience what that means. And God through those circumstances is calling us to give up our ways to take on His. He is speaking through the everyday conditions of your life and mine, if we but have ears to hear and hearts to understand.

If our way is hard and we cannot see how it is going to work out for good, it is time to trust. "In returning and rest you shall be saved; in quietness and trust shall be your strength" (v. 15). If our way is smooth and pleasant, let it be a reminder of how greatly we are loved, and let it spur us on to more faithful obedience to the Lord.

> Halts by me that footfall:
> Is my gloom, after all,
> Shade of His hand, outstretched caressingly!
> *(Hound of Heaven, F. Thompson, 1859-1907)*

A Prayer: *Lord, give me eyes to see You and ears to hear what You are saying through the circumstances of my life. I thank You that You are with me in them, and that the darkness in them is "the shade of Your hand, outstretched caressingly." In Jesus' Name. Amen.*

1. Where in your circumstances of life has God been speaking to you?

2. What have you done about it?

Week 4, Day 7

Listening to Others

Daily Reading: Ephesians 4:15-32

Rather speaking the truth in love, we are to grow up in every way into him who is the head, into Christ (v. 15).

This week we have been thinking about hearing God in various ways. One of the hardest ways for most of us is to hear Him through other people. Yet we are told very clearly here to "speak the truth in love" to one another. Down further on, Paul tells us, "Let everyone speak the truth with his neighbor" (v. 25).

Robert Burns, the Scottish poet, has a little verse which says, "O would some Power the giftie gie us, to see oursel's as others see us." As a matter of fact, Christians have been given that "giftie." If we are truthful with one another, we cannot only see ourselves as others see us, we can begin to get a better view of ourselves as God sees us.

We know, or we should know, what the Prophet Jeremiah said about the human heart—about our own hearts: "The heart is deceitful above all things, and desperately corrupt; who can understand it!" (Jeremiah 17:9). Our hearts tell us all that we are good, that we mean well, that we are right. But others often tell us a different story. If we will but listen to those who speak to us—even if we think they are speaking out of their own sin—God will honor that, and we will begin to get a different and healing view of ourselves. That is the word of testimony of many people who have subjected themselves to the discipline of listening to others.

Pride and ego can build a wonderful but false image of ourselves to ourselves. The truth begins to tear down and destroy that image. It is painful, but it is worth it, because in its place, God offers us freedom from having to keep up that false image, freedom from having to feed the monster ego which is never satisfied, and the joy of simply being in Him.

"A man who flatters his neighbor spreads a net for his feet" (Proverbs 29:5). Do we seek flattery or truth? Do we speak the truth in love, or do we spread nets for the feet of friends?

A Prayer: *Spirit of truth, give me a love for thee.*
Let me not despise nor reject thee in any guise.
Let me welcome and receive thee and be wise.
In Jesus' Name, Amen.

1. What areas are there in your life in which you need to grow up?

2. What steps can you take?

Week Review

Listening is often harder than speaking. It is especially true if God is speaking what you do not want to hear.

1. Where is God speaking to you and how is He speaking?

2. Do you hear God when He is telling you when you are disobedient?

3. Describe one situation where you believe you heard God and you took action as a result.

SPIRITUAL JOURNAL

Hearing God is dependent upon one condition—the desire to be obedient to Him.

M. Cay & M. Judy

The Blessing of Obedience

"He who has my commandments and keeps them, he it is who loves me; and he who loves me will be loved by my Father, and I will love him and manifest myself to him."

John 14:21

A Blessing and a Curse

Daily Reading: Deuteronomy 11:8-32

Behold, I set before you this day a blessing and a curse; the blessing if you obey the commandments of the Lord your God, which I command you this day, and the curse, if you do not obey the commandments of the Lord your God, but turn aside from the way which I command you this day, to go after other gods which you have not known. (vv. 26-28)

Obedience brings blessing—obedience to God, that is, instead of obedience to "other gods." Our Scripture makes very plain that two ways are set before us—God's way and the way of "other gods." The one path is the path to blessing. The other is the path to ruin. Israel is being challenged to "choose life."

We all know that children are not naturally obedient. Their nature is to do what they like, and it is with careful (sometimes painful) training that they learn that obeying mother and father brings more satisfaction than getting away with whatever they want to do. As parents, we know, too, how difficult it is to be consistent in requiring obedience for the sake of the children.

God is not an unreasonable tyrant. He has not so constructed His world that He requires obedience for capricious reasons. He requires obedience because of His love. Everything that He asks of us is grounded in His love for us. We should always look at the requirement of obedience in that light, even though obedience may seem less rewarding in the short run than disobedience! The *truth* is here: Blessing, if we obey the commandments of the Lord. It is built into the very nature of things.

The sad story of Israel throughout the Old Testament is the story of people who did not learn to be obedient and suffered the consequences. God did not abandon them, and still sent words of hope and promise, but what a lot of grief and suffering they could have been spared had they learned to be obedient.

All of us are *still* learning. We are not yet perfected in obedience. Only One was perfectly obedient—Jesus our Lord. But the same blessing promised of old still holds—if we will set our wills to be obedient. Start where you can! Keep at it! Don't give up! The blessing is worth it.

A Prayer: *Great and many are the blessings I have already received from You, O Lord. I pray for the grace of an obedient spirit, in Jesus' Name. Amen.*

1. Where are you discovering the blessing of obedience in your life?

If You Love Me

Daily Reading: John 14:15-31

If you love Me, you will keep My commandments. (v. 15)

This is a strong and disturbing verse. It clearly says that obedience is the proof of love and the expression of love. In another place, Jesus says, "Why do you call me Lord, Lord, and do not do the things that I say?" (Luke 6:46)

"Yes, Lord, you know that I love you!" That is what Peter said to Jesus when they met after the resurrection. It was not spoken hastily or lightly—for Peter remembered with shame and sorrow how he had deserted the Lord after vowing that he would give his life and die for Him if necessary. But Peter could only say in spite of all he had done, in spite of all he had not done, "Lord, you know all things. You know that I love you."

Jesus gives us this strong and disturbing word because we need it. Self-love is so strong that unless we are pulled up short, it can easily take over and crowd out our love for Him. Like the weeds in the parable of the sower, "the cares of the world, and the delight in riches, and the desire for other things, enter in, and choke the word and it proves unfruitful." (Mark 4:19)

We cannot, in and of ourselves, love Him. That is His gift to us. With St Paul, we must admit that without Jesus Christ and the work of the Holy Spirit within, we are locked in a nature that is totally self-oriented and self-concerned, often confounding us with our own contradictions! But, if He has given us grace to love Him, then He will give more grace. Obedience brings added grace, and we can move from strength to strength.

> Jesus, what didst thou find in me
> That thou hast dealt so lovingly!
> How great the joy that thou hast brought!
> So far exceeding hope or thought!
> Jesus my Lord, I thee adore:
> O make me love thee more and more!
>
> *(Henry Collins, 1854)*

A Prayer: *Make us of quick and tender conscience, O Lord; that understanding, we may obey every word of Thine this day, and discerning, may follow every suggestion of Thine indwelling Spirit. Speak, Lord, for Thy servant heareth; through Jesus Christ our Lord. Amen.* *(Christina G. Rossetti, 1830)*

1. How does your self-love express itself?

2. How can you break out of self-centeredness?

If You Keep My Commandments

Daily Reading: John 15:1-11

If you keep My commandments, you will abide in My love, just as I have kept My Father's commandments and abide in His love. (v. 10)

Yesterday we thought about obedience as the proof and acid test of our love for Jesus. Today's scripture turns the subject around, and reminds us of the promise of what obedience will bring.

"You will abide in My love." What does it mean to abide in His love? It means to be one in spirit with all that He is and all He is doing. It means to live in the daily, moment-by-moment blessing of His grace and favor in our lives.

Perhaps you have experienced a small taste of this with another human being. You loved that person, and as long as you and the other person were in unity of spirit, there was an atmosphere of freedom and trust between you. You wanted to please the other because you loved, and you were pleased by the other because you were loved by him or her.

This is an inadequate but helpful picture of what He is saying. Breaking the commandments brings about disjuncture, a fracturing of the relationship. We are injured by our own disobedience, and our Lord suffers, too. Otherwise, we had no part in His crucifixion and death, if our sins do not really hurt. And so, when we willfully disobey, we are not "abiding in His love." That does not mean that He ceases to love us; it does not even mean that we have ceased to love Him. But it does mean that the fellowship and oneness are broken, and all the blessing that flowed to us from that oneness is cut off, waiting to be restored and renewed.

Jesus felt that abiding in His Father's love was worth everything that obedience cost. He even endured the cross, despising the shame. He promises no less for us; if we obey, the blessing of abiding in His love will be worth everything it costs!

A Prayer: I rest upon thy word; the promise is for me;
My succor and salvation, Lord, shall surely come from thee.
But let me still abide, nor from my hope remove,
Till thou my patient spirit guide into thy perfect love. Amen.

(Charles Wesley, 1742)

1. Have you seen any place in your life recently when you have been willfully disobedient? Where?

2. What were the results?

Slaves of the One You Obey

Daily Reading: Romans 6:12-23

Do you not know that if you yield yourselves to any one as obedient slaves, you are slaves of the one whom you obey, either of sin, which leads to death or of obedience, which leads to righteousness? (v. 16)

Paul here in this sixth chapter of Romans develops further the intimate, almost organic, relationship between obedience and abiding in Christ.

The figure of speech he uses is that of slave. We cannot be absolutely free—even though we may fool ourselves that we *are* free when we do as we please. The truth is, that we are in that very moment (if what we please is disobedience!), yielding ourselves as *slaves* of sin! We can choose our master, but it will be one or the other—sin or Christ.

That puts the matter quite plainly: we choose who is going to have dominion over us. Once we had no choice—our nature took care of that, as members of Adam's fallen race. But Jesus Christ entered our race, took our human nature upon Himself, lived a life of perfect obedience and died in our place, in order that sin need not have dominion over us any more. He is the Key of David who unlocks the prisonhouse of our old self-bondage. With Him, we can become "slaves of obedience," which Paul says leads to righteousness.

Someone may ask, "What kind of a choice is that—just a choice of masters?" Yet to answer it, we have only to look back at where the other kind of slavery—slavery to sin—took us; or where it takes others whom we know and love. Becoming obedient does not mean that we lose the temptation to choose sin, nor does it mean that we have entered a new kind of bondage. For with obedience comes life, grace, peace and joy. Against these, who can complain?

A Prayer: *O God, who art the author of peace and lover of concord, in knowledge of Whom standeth our eternal life, whose service is perfect freedom, defend us thy humble servants in all assaults of our enemies; that we, surely trusting in thy defense, may not fear the power of any adversaries, through the might of Jesus Christ our Lord. Amen.*

(Service of Daily Morning Prayer, Book of Common Prayer, Italics added.)

1. How do you feel about not having your own way?

2. What do you do with how you feel?

Week 5, Day 5

I Was Not Disobedient to the Heavenly Vision

Daily Reading: Acts 26:1-32

Wherefore, O King Agrippa, I was not disobedient to the heavenly vision. (v. 19)

This week we are thinking about the blessing of obedience and the importance of obedience. As members of a 3D group, we are asked to indicate on our Food Sheets when and how we have been "disobedient" in the food discipline. It may seem a small thing, but it is important. Jesus said, "He who is faithful in a very little is faithful also in much." (Luke 16:10) Let us try to see our disobedience in God's perspective!

But today's scripture speaks of another dimension of obedience. Paul's obedience "to the heavenly vision" was an indispensable element in his faithfulness to Jesus Christ. It was not simply a matter of doing right things, avoiding wrong things— as it had been in the days when he was a practicing Pharisee. Now his obedience included faithfulness to the vision the Lord had given him. When we think back to the fruit of that obedience (he was the first great Christian missionary!), it is impossible to overestimate its blessing. His letters to churches and individuals make up some of the most valuable and helpful portions of the Holy Scriptures, so that even today, our debt to him is immeasurable.

Are we obedient to our "heavenly vision"? Have you had given to you some inspiration, some goal, some worthy thing to do, which you believed came from God? Treasure it, and be faithful to it. "Where there is no vision, the people perish." (Proverbs 29:18) Without this long-range goal toward which we can strive and move, life can mire in the concerns of the moment, and our spiritual muscles can become flaccid.

A Prayer: *O Lord God, when Thou givest to Thy servants to endeavor any great matter, grant us also to know that it is not the beginning but the continuing of the same until it be thoroughly finished which yieldeth the true glory. Amen.*

(Sir Francis Drake, 1540-1596)

1. List ways you have sought to be obedient this week.

2. What were the results?

Be Subject to One Another

Daily Reading: Ephesians 5:1-33

Be subject to one another out of reverence for Christ. (v. 21)

Perhaps the hardest part of obedience is learning to subject our wills to the will of another. None of us likes to be told what to do! We fear that to subject ourselves to another will mean the loss of freedom and possible annihilation of our own personalities.

Yet we are clearly instructed: "Be subject to one another out of reverence for Christ." Strength—physical or psychological—should not be the determining factor as to whose way prevails. The strong should serve the weak, and those who seem weak are often psychologically stronger than the physically strong! And so Paul instructs wives to be subject to their husbands "as to the Lord," and husbands to lay down their lives (including their own "rights") as Christ laid down His life for the Church. No one, then, would be lording it over anyone else, for there would be a mutual subjection to one another. In the Gospels we read Jesus' words: "The kings of the Gentiles exercise lordship over them, and those in authority over them are called benefactors. But not so with you; rather let the greatest among you become as the youngest, and the leader as one who serves." (Luke 22:25,26)

If we are subjecting ourselves to one another out of reverence for Christ, this means that we are hearing what Jesus has to say to us through another person. If we become suspicious enough of our own willful tendencies, we will not be so afraid to put down our own will to do what someone else suggests, when we know that they are not leading us into anything sinful or wrong. It is not an easy assignment. But this attitude is essential if we are to "walk in love, as Christ loved us." (v. 2) Remember that He said He came, not to do His own will, but the will of Him who sent Him. This, too, should be our goal in being subject to one another out of reverence for Christ.

A Prayer Thought: *If there be any good in thee, believe that this is much more in others—that so though mayest preserve humility within thee.*

(Thomas a Kempis)

1. Note any other things the Lord has shown you about obedience.

2. What fear do you have about being obedient to others?

Faith Without Works

Daily Reading: James 2:8-26

So faith by itself, if it has no works, is dead. (v. 17)

We have thought about obedience as the path to blessing, as a proof of our love for God, as underwritten by God's promises of His abiding presence. We have considered the option of being slaves to sin and death or to obedience and life, and noted that the long-range vision as well as the duty of the moment demands our faithful obedience. We have thought about the problem of subjecting ourselves to do what another person tells us or wants us to do.

Today's scripture was written with people in mind who insisted that faith alone was all they needed, and who disregarded the necessity of obedience to the truth. James is greatly concerned that we see the deception of such thinking, and that where faith is alive, works (read "obedience") follow. Doing good things is not the way to God, but neither is "head belief" without works that demonstrate the sincerity of one's faith.

This brings us back to the basic struggle we all face as Christians. It is the struggle between self, in all its devious ways of deception, and the call to obedience, with its disarming simplicity. All of us face this struggle every day, and as we seek to be faithful in simple obediences, we find that we understand better the nature of the struggle going on within.

Thank God for a living faith that can produce obedience as its fruit! Let us pray daily for an increase of *that* faith!

A Prayer Thought: *Pray Him to give you what Scripture calls "an honest and good heart," or "a perfect heart," and, without waiting, begin at once to obey Him with the best heart you have. Any obedience is better than none.*

You have to seek His face; obedience is the only way of seeing Him. All your duties are obediences. To do what He bids is to obey Him, and to obey Him is to approach Him. (John Henry Cardinal Newman, 1801-1890)

1. Describe any struggle that might have gone on within you this week between self and the call of obedience.

Week Review

You have been learning about obedience. It is not always easy. The disciplines may sometimes seem to be overwhelming. We trust you are feeling free enough to talk about any discouragement you might have in your group.

1. Are you discouraged about your weight loss? If so, have you been honest about your feelings to allow God to change your heart? Sometimes we are blessed in a different way than we had in mind.

2. What other areas in your life do you find difficult in being obedient?

SPIRITUAL JOURNAL

If you'll only be obedient, He'll turn everything within you to His way.

M. Cay & M. Judy

Nobody Tells Me What to Do! (Rebellion)

"Behold, to obey is better than sacrifice, and to hearken than the fat of rams. For rebellion is as the sin of witchcraft, and stubbornness is as iniquity and idolatry."
I Samuel 15:22b,23 (KJV)

Rebellion Is As the Sin of Witchcraft

Daily Reading: I Samuel 15

For rebellion is as the sin of divination, and stubbornness is as iniquity and idolatry. (v. 23a)

Saul put his own judgment ahead of God's clear command. He reasoned that since Agag was king, he should not be destroyed along with other Ammonites. He reasoned that it would be a shame to kill the good sheep, oxen, fatlings and lambs (as he had been instructed to do). So when Samuel arrived at Gilgal, Saul confidently exclaimed, "I have performed the commandment of the Lord." "What then is this bleating of the sheep in my ears, and the lowing of the oxen which I hear!" asked Samuel. Saul's explanation was to no avail. His reasoning did not matter. What mattered was obedience to the clear command of the Lord. "Why did you not obey the voice of the Lord?" Samuel persisted. And Saul then did a very interesting thing (not at all unlike the things we do when we are confronted with our wrong). He said, "I have obeyed. . . . I have gone on the mission. . . . I have brought Agag. . . . I have destroyed. . . . But the people. . . ." In order to excuse his own disobedience, he put the blame "on the people."

There is an important lesson for us all in this passage. The inner rebellion against whatever God is requiring of us leads to all kinds of reasoning, rationalization, and excuse-making. It may fool us for awhile. But it does not fool God. There has to be a reckoning time, and the spirit of rebellion within must be dealt with. Better that it be dealt with early, before it has time to do its destructive work in us and in others around us. Equating it with witchcraft or divination (a kind of fortune-telling) is intended to show us the depth of its wickedness, so that we may turn from it with abhorrence.

A Prayer: *O our God, bestow upon us such confidence, such peace, such happiness in Thee, that Thy will may always be dearer to us than our own will, and Thy pleasure than our own pleasure. All that Thou givest is Thy free gift to us, and all that Thou takest away is Thy grace to us. Be Thou thanked for all, praised for all, loved for all; through Jesus Christ our Lord. Amen.*

(Christina G. Rossetti, 1830-1894)

1. This very clear picture of Saul's disobedience can speak to us. Where have you seen that you blame others to excuse yourself?

2. Where have you rationalized your decisions or your behavior?

A Stubborn and Rebellious Generation

Daily Reading: Psalm 78:1-20

And that they should not be like their fathers, a stubborn and rebellious generation whose heart was not steadfast, whose spirit was not faithful to God. (v. 8)

The Psalmist relates here a parable, "a dark saying from of old, that he had heard from 'our fathers'." It was a sad but glorious story of God's faithfulness and Israel's rebellion. This long Psalm becomes a kind of "Reader's Digest" history of Israel, citing the wonderful deliverances of God and the sad tendency of the people to turn away from Him.

As we read it, however, we are aware that it is more than the story of an ancient people and their God. It is also the story of our rebellion and of God's judgments and mercies. For we know that He is the same, yesterday, today and for ever.

What did God do to meet this rebellion? "He established a testimony in Jacob and appointed a law in Israel." (v. 5) That was His first move, to set up the evidence of His merciful deliverance (the testimony) and what He required of those who would be His people.

Paul discusses their failure to keep the law, and concludes that the Law declares us all guilty before God-Jew and Gentile alike-so that we are all in need of His mercy and forgiveness.

But see here the compassion of God, and His infinite patience with His chosen people. His manna in the wilderness and the water from the rock should have been ample testimony of His care.

What about the testimony, the witness of God's mercy in your life and mine? Do we ignore it, or do we let it work life in us? That is the question. For He has established a testimony, a record of loving deeds for us as surely as He did for Israel of old!

A Prayer: *Grant to us, Lord, we beseech thee, the spirit to think and do always such things as are right; that we, who cannot do any thing that is good without thee, may by thee be enabled to live according to thy will; through Jesus Christ our Lord. Amen.*

(Collect for the 9th Sunday after Trinity, Book of Common Prayer)

1. Against what specific things do you find yourself rebelling?

2. How can you cooperate with God in your daily life in order that you can choose God's will?

Yet They Rebelled

Daily Reading: Psalm 78:32-72

Yet they tested and rebelled against the Most High God, and did not observe His testimonies, but turned away and acted treacherously like their fathers. (vv. 56,57a)

The latter part of this Psalm catalogues the folly of continued rebellion in the face of all God's dealings. His "destroying visitations" seemed to produce a temporary return to God. "When he slew them, they sought for him; they repented and sought God earnestly." (v. 34) But these returns were short-lived, and soon the pull of the old ways was stronger than their fear of God's judgments.

Does that sound familiar? Do we not do the same-return under affliction, and find the mercy freeflowing, and then find that our self-will and old habits pull strongly against what we know to be the will of God?

Our rebellious nature is something we have to recognize. Otherwise we will be like Saul at Gilgal, affirming that we have done everything the Lord wants us to do, when in reality we are doing what we want to do. That is one of the reasons why it is important to let others have some authority in our lives, permission to tell us what to do in one or another area. Simply allowing the leaders to give us the amount of food exchanges allowed each day can be an important step in conquering this inner rebellion. Submitting to the other disciplines can be of further help.

Israel was finally carried away, never to be seen again as a result of her rebellion. Only little Judah remained to carry on the testimony of God. Israel stands as a permanent warning to us of the effect of persistent rebellion against a Holy God.

> Perverse and foolish oft I strayed,
> And yet in love He sought me,
> And on His shoulder gently laid
> And home rejoicing brought me.
> *Henry Baker, 1868 (based on Psalm 23)*

A Prayer: *I know, O Lord, and do with all humility acknowledge myself as an object altogether unworthy of Thy love; but sure I am, Thou art an object altogether worthy of mine. Do Thou then impart to me some of that excellence, and that shall supply my own lack of worth. Help me to cease from sin according to Thy will, that I may be capable of doing Thee service according to my duty.*

(St Augustine, 254-430, abridged)

1. Self-will and old habits often rob us of spiritual gains. How can we stand against these?

2. How can you begin to establish new habits?

Do Not Harden Your Hearts

Daily Reading: Hebrews 3

But exhort one another every day, as long as it is called "today," that none of you may be hardened by the deceitfulness of sin. (v. 13)

One commentator on these verses says, "Tomorrow is the day when idle men and fools repent. Tomorrow is Satan's today; he cares not what resolutions you form, if only you fix them for tomorrow."

Whenever we are called on to make any forward progress in our life of personal discipline and obedience, the tempter whispers, "This one time won't matter that much." Whenever we are tempted to disobey or ignore one of the disciplines, the same thing comes into our minds. In this way, we are hardened by "the deceitfulness of sin." The old pattern is continued, becoming fixed in a kind of "conditioned response" to a given situation. Something happens that makes us feel sorry for ourselves, or we get angry or resentful, we are disappointed, or actually hurt or put down by someone else. In such a case, look out! The tempter will come and whisper, "You can resume your discipline tomorrow!"

It is very important that we see this part of human nature, and guard ourselves against it. "Exhort one another every day," says the writer of Hebrews. Exhort yourself, and help anyone else whom you have responsibility for-and be willing to ask for help from fellow group members when the temptation comes to ignore or give up the disciplines!

The hardened heart through the deceitfulness of sin only sets us up for more painful situations later on. Since God is working with us to bring us more fully into conformity with His will, we must expect that He will keep on working, in many and various ways, to soften our hearts and to clarify our vision, so that we be not blinded with the deceitfulness of sin.

A Prayer Thought: *"Blake has told us that Satan is the god of things that are not, 'the traveller's dream under the hill.' He is the god of the rainbow in the next field but one, in seeking whom men miss the true God in the meadow where they stand."* (Arthur Clutton-Brock)

A Prayer: *Make and keep my heart soft, O Lord, and sensitive to the moving of Your Holy Spirit. In Jesus' Name. Amen.*

1. What are you tempted to do when you are sorry for yourself, angry or resentful?

2. Where this week have you been willing to ask for help and be needy when you are finding the disciplines difficult or you are feeling "stuck" somewhere?

I Have Rebelled

Daily Reading: Lamentations 1

The Lord is in the right, for I have rebelled against His word. (v. 18a)

Lamentations is a book of tragic songs, sung by the prophet Jeremiah as he saw Judah and Jerusalem being destroyed and carried away captive. In it we see the grief and anguish of the prophet's heart as Jerusalem reaps the reward of her rebellion. Here in the first chapter, Jeremiah speaks for Jerusalem, confessing her sin and waiting for the mercy of God.

All this week we are thinking about the reality of rebellion in the human race, and of our own specific part in it. Rebellion demands punishment on God's part if He is to remain Lord of His own universe. "The Lord is in the right." The rebel is in the wrong. Man cannot excuse his uprising against God's government, and we cannot excuse our own rebellion against what we know God requires of us. What is sown is reaped, and the effects can be heartbreaking.

D. L. Moody is reported to have said once to a group of students, "Don't forget that 'whatsoever a man soweth, that shall he also reap.' You have got to reap what you sow. Do you ask, 'If I repent and God forgives me, will I still have to reap?' Yes, you will; nothing can change that law. But if you repent, God will help you in the hard work of reaping."

It should neither surprise us nor dismay us when we see the results of our rebellion displayed in our life situations, our relationships, our children, and so on. That is no time for despair, the throwing up of hands and giving up. Instead, we can say, "The Lord is in the right, for I have rebelled against His word." We can begin to cooperate with Him, so that He can bring good out of evil, and can help us "in the hard work of reaping." He is using it all for good and for His glory, and that should be a tremendous word of hope and encouragement to any of us!

A Prayer: *Lord, open my eyes to see the true nature of rebellion before too many seeds are sown for a sad harvest. And anything that I must walk through because of past rebellion, do be with me, and give me grace to see Your loving hand. In Jesus' Name. Amen.*

1. Where have you come to see you have sought to excuse your rebellion?

2. Rather than despair, where do you see you can cooperate with God to bring blessing out of your disobedience?

The Rebellion of Korah

Daily Reading: Numbers 16

Therefore it is against the Lord that you and all your company have gathered together; what is Aaron that you murmur against him? (v. 11)

The rebellion of Korah and his followers stands as an extreme and graphic example and warning to Israel and to all of us against the sin of rebellion. A conspiracy had been formed and two hundred and fifty men were involved in it, challenging the leadership of Moses and Aaron. Here are some thoughts for our meditation:

First, their rebellion was rooted in jealousy. When we find ourselves inwardly resisting or resenting those in places of leadership, we should be suspicious of our own motivation. Jealousy is an insidious sin, and it quickly spreads, feeding on small dissatisfactions and resulting at times in major crises. More harm is done to Christian fellowship by this sin than any other.

Second, the rebellion was aided by back-biting. The dictionary defines back-biting as "saying mean and spiteful things about a person who is absent." Jealousy uses back-biting in order to do its destructive work. Rebellion could not become conspiracy without it.

Third, those who engaged in rebellion were the ones who were ultimately harmed. God has pledged Himself to protect and defend His work. "Lo, I am with you always," said Jesus, "even to the close of the age." But if we place ourselves, even unwittingly, against what God is doing, then we endanger our own interests. In every group, church, congregation, or fellowship, it is important to guard ourselves against the spirit of rebellion; every discipline carries with it the temptation to resist and rebel. So let us behave wisely in the light of what we are seeing.

A Prayer: *O merciful God, bless Thy people throughout all the world, and all who love Thee in sincerity, although they follow not with us in all things. Heal all strife, division, and discord, and make us all Thine in willing devotion as we are all Thine by redemption and grace; for the sake of Jesus Christ our Lord. Amen.*
(H. W. Turner, 19th century)

1. Prayerfully go over your life and make a list of people in leadership or authority of whom you have been jealous.

2. Go over the list and confess this jealousy to the Lord, accept the forgiveness of God and go on rejoicing and change!

The Fruit of Rebellion

Daily Reading: Romans 1:18-32

Therefore God gave them up in the lusts of their hearts to impurity, to the dishonoring of their bodies among themselves, because they exchanged the truth about God for a lie, and worshipped and served the creature rather than the creator, who is blessed forever! Amen. (vv. 24,25)

This section has been aptly referred to as the darkest description of human nature in the Bible. Paul is concerned here to shock us with the ultimate direction in which rebellion takes us. He wants us to be sickened by the description of men and women abandoned to what is in them apart from the grace of God.

We are confronted here with the terrible wrath of God which has been revealed from heaven against all sin—small and great. Everywhere men's consciences register His wrath, until by continually rebelling against Him, the conscience becomes so seared and deadened that it can no longer register God's wrath, and so are given up by God to whatever is in the heart. "Willful resistance of light," says David Brown, "has a retributive tendency to blind the moral perceptions and weaken the capacity to apprehend and approve of truth and goodness; and thus is the soul prepared to surrender itself, to an indefinite extent, to error and sin." The key term is "willful resistance to light." We are not responsible for what we have not been taught. "The times of this ignorance God winked at," says Acts 17:30, "but now commands men everywhere to repent." In other words, we are morally and spiritually responsible for the light we are given. This is especially important when we are hearing it from someone else, and do not like what we are hearing. Instead of "willful resistance to light," we should struggle against ourselves to receive the light within, that knowing where we are wrong, where we need to change, where we need to repent, we can step further in the light, and manifest more of Jesus' likeness.

The fruit of rebellion, when God gives a person up to the lusts of the heart, is frightening indeed. Let it warn us away from its earlier motions.

A Prayer: *Make us of quick and tender conscience, O Lord; that understanding, we may obey every word of Thine this day, and discerning, may follow every suggestion of Thine indwelling Spirit. Speak, Lord, for Thy servant heareth; through Jesus Christ our Lord.* (Christina G. Rosetti, 1830-94)

1. Note anything else the Lord has shown you about rebellion.

Week Review

When we hear the word "rebellion," we think of extremely "bad" behavior—something easily recognized. In reality, rebellion is simply not being willing to be obedient.

Rebellion can also be very subtle, especially when you think you have an excuse to be disobedient.

1. Think about those specific places in 3D where you are rebellious, and do you need any help?

2. Have you discovered any habit patterns that encourage your rebellion?

3. What are you putting off "until tomorrow"?

4. How do you overcome rebellion?

SPIRITUAL JOURNAL

How can a sovereign God rule and reign in a "temple" that already has a ruler called self?

M. Cay & M. Judy

"Those Whom I Love I Reprove" (Correction)

"For the Lord disciplines him whom He loves, and chastises every son whom He receives."

Hebrews 12:6

Bearing the Burden of Correction

Daily Reading: Galatians 6:1-10

Brethren, if a man is overtaken in any trespass, you who are spiritual should restore him in a spirit of gentleness . . . . Bear one another's burdens, and so fulfill the law of Christ. (vv. 1,2)

It comes as a distinct surprise to many Christians that they may have some obligation to correct other Christians! This is so foreign to the experience most of us have had in the Church that it may seem to be a new or strange teaching. Actually, the "new and strange teaching" is the idea that has crept into Christianity that we do not have responsibility for dealing with one another's faults.

If a person is in a fault or "trespass," how can he or she be "restored" unless the trespass is talked about? And if it is talked about, it must be done lovingly but in the spirit of truth and frankness. Such a thing is almost unthinkable in today's church, except where small groups of people covenant together to give and receive correction one of another. It may seem very risky, and certainly no one is going to enjoy (for the moment) receiving correction by others. But what it can do, when it is carefully and lovingly done, is to open up a depth of caring Christian fellowship which can be the greatest blessing imaginable.

The "burden" of speaking correction to a brother or sister in Christ means that we feel the risk of being rejected by that person if we tell them the truth. That burden, however, can open the way to forgiveness, freedom, and a new joy when the other person has "been restored."

Each person has to bear his or her own load, too. That means (at least in part) that when we receive correction from others—wife, husband, employer, friend, parent, etc.—we can and must "bear" it, in order to become free of false estimates of ourselves. The way is very clear, and the blessings are abundant, if we are willing to walk in it.

The 3D experience is a tiny beginning at this kind of sharing. Treasure it and pray that the Holy Spirit will prepare you for whatever else He has in mind for your growth in Christ.

1. During this week you will find that some people are easier for you to be honest with than others. Who is the hardest for you, and why?

But When I Saw They Were Not Straightforward

Daily Reading: Galatians 2

But when Cephas came to Antioch I opposed him to his face, because he stood condemned. (v. 11)

Cephas is Peter. Apparently Peter had difficulty at this point in his life in living out what he really believed in the face of opposition. He cared what other people thought about him! When he came to Antioch, at first he mingled with the non-Jewish Christians and ate with them as equals. Then came "certain men from James," representing a group who felt that all Christians should be circumcised and follow the Jewish rites. It had become quite a point of controversy in the Jerusalem church, and they were concerned when they heard that Paul and Barnabas were not requiring Gentiles to become Jewish proselytes when they became Christians.

Paul himself had been the strictest kind of Jew, and he knew from personal experience what observing the Law meant. He also knew that God had thrown open the door of the Kingdom to all-to the Jew first and also to the Gentile! And when Peter, fearing criticism from the delegation from Jerusalem and the "folks back home," jumped up from the Gentile table and went over to a table made up of Jews only, Paul "opposed him to his face."

This is a good example of how correction worked in the early church. The concern for truth was greater than the concern for personal feelings. That, of course, can be an excuse for erupting one's feelings out of jealousy, anger, hurt feelings, and other motives, if we are not concerned with the other aspects of our fellowship: receiving as well as giving correction, and maintaining the "unity of the spirit in the bond of peace."

But the point is important. Christians must be willing to speak when another Christian is in the wrong. Usually it is wise to have a third person (see Matthew 18:16) when speaking to someone about a fault or trespass.

A Prayer: *Lord, make me quick to hear a word of reproof, and willing to speak the truth to my brothers and sisters as led by Your Holy Spirit. Above all, help me to see myself, first, as "the chief of sinners," so that my self-righteousness will not be a stumbling-block. In Jesus' Name. Amen.*

1. What do you really care more about-the concern to be honest, or what other people think? Why?

Let Everyone Speak the Truth

Daily Reading: Ephesians 4

Therefore putting away falsehood, let every one speak the truth with his neighbor, for we are members one of another. (v. 25)

As we are considering the subject of correction (or reproof), it is well to ask the Lord wherein we are dishonest in our relationships with fellow Christians. Do we flatter insincerely? Do we change the facts to make them a little more acceptable when repeating something to another? Do we pretend to approve of some attitude which we know to be wrong and hurtful? Do we indulge in repeating hearsay and gossip which does no good, and serves to divide the fellowship? Do we listen to gossip, even if we do not repeat it? And if so, do we realize that listening makes us as guilty as speaking it?

The young church at Ephesus was a church in a hostile environment. At this time Christians were often ostracized and shunned for their faith. Paul himself writes the letter from prison. "I therefore, a prisoner for the Lord, beg you to lead a life worthy of the calling to which you have been called." (v. 1) If that young fellowship did not learn to be *truthful* within itself, it would have no inner strength to stand against the forces outside.

Today, we are yet again in great need of the spiritual buttressing received when Christians speak the truth to one another in love. It is a freeing experience. We truly cannot know ourselves without the help of others who will speak the truth to us.

"Truth is the secret of eloquence and of virtue, the basis of moral authority; it is the highest summit of art and of life."   (Henri-Frederic Amiel, Journal, 1883)

A Prayer: *Almighty God, Who hast sent the Spirit of truth unto us to guide us into all truth, so rule our lives by Thy power, that we may be truthful in word, deed, and thought. O keep us, most merciful Saviour, with thy gracious protection, so that no fear or hope may ever make us false in act or speech; and bring us all to the perfect freedom of thy truth; through Jesus Christ our Lord. Amen.*

(Bishop Westcott, 1825, abridged)

1. Have you seen any places that you flatter insincerely or change the facts to make them more acceptable? Where?

2. Where this week have you been willing to speak the truth with your neighbor (or family)?

Week 7, Day 4

Have I Become Your Enemy?

Daily Reading: Galatians 4:8-31

Have I then become your enemy by telling you the truth? (v. 16)

The truth is, that in our feelings this is exactly what happens when someone speaks unpleasant truth to us. We often do not even recognize it as truth. It seems like criticism, condemnation, even rejection. Our reaction, then, is hurt, anger, self-defense! We are attacked and the person speaking is the enemy.

Paul knew that this was probably the way the Galatian Christians were reacting to his rebuke. The whole letter is a stern and loving rebuke of a man who had poured out his life to give these people the Good News of Jesus Christ! Now he saw them in danger of selling their spiritual birthright for a mess of legal pottage, and he was angry! He was angry at those who had come into the flock of new Christians and upset their faith, and he was appalled at the Galatians for being so gullible. But there is power in truth. There is light and healing in it. When it is spoken, the hearer has the opportunity of choosing to believe it, even though feelings may go in exactly the opposite direction. After all, if we are ruled by our feelings, none of us is very stable! So we can choose to give up considering the person who speaks to us as "the enemy." We can choose to put down our defenses, and pray for even a small corner of agreement, where we can "agree with our adversary quickly." In this way, we treat the person as a friend and helper instead of an enemy, and once we have given up the self-righteous defense mechanism all of us have, we can begin to come into greater light and understanding, repentance and freedom. It is a secret too few of us know and fully appreciate, but one which saints and heroes of faith have long treasured. It allows the cross to work on our old nature, as the truth convicts and sets us free.

> Truth being truth,
> Tell it and shame the devil.
>
> *(Robert Browning)*

A Prayer: *Help me the slow of heart to move, by some clear, winning word of love. Teach me the wayward feet to stay, and guide them in the homeward way. Amen.* *(Washington Gladden, 1879)*

1. Is there someone specific you resist when they speak to you? Who? Why?

2. Where have you allowed the truth spoken to you set you free and help you change?

Respect Those . . . Who Admonish You

Daily Reading: I Thessalonians 5

But we beseech you, brethren, to respect those who labor among you and are over you in the Lord and admonish you, and to esteem them very highly in love because of their work. (vv. 12,13a)

Admonish. 1a. To indicate duties or obligations to. b. to express warning or disapproval to, especially gently, earnestly and solicitously. 2. to give friendly, earnest advice or encouragement.

The word comes from the word meaning "to warn." Those who admonish us are those who warn us of possible or real dangers in our lives if we follow certain courses of action.

What place has admonishment in our lives as Christians, and as 3D members? Do you ever feel a warning for someone else who is going through a difficult time and asks for help? Do you expose your own struggle and temptation, so that others may give you "friendly, earnest advice or encouragement"?

Group leaders, pastors, perhaps others, do have a responsibility for those entrusted to their care, to give such help as they can. *All* of us without exception, high or low, need to be admonished from time to time. We have seen Paul admonishing Peter. We read many examples of it in the New Testament. To avoid being admonished is to run the danger of leaning on our own understanding and placing ourselves above all others. Such an attitude breaks fellowship and separates us from our families and other members of the Body of Christ.

A Prayer: *Lord Jesus, Yours is the most humble of hearts; I confess that by nature I am inclined to haughtiness and that my heart's evil spirit is poisoned by pride, the root of all sin. Grant me true lowliness so that I may imitate Your holy humility, becoming like a child. Amen.* (Johann Arndt, c. 1600)

1. What are some of the ways God has admonished you?

2. Where have you cared enough for people to lovingly and mercifully admonish them?

The Rebuke of the Wise

Daily Reading: Ecclesiastes 7:1-20

It is better for a man to hear the rebuke of the wise than to hear the song of fools. (v. 5)

By nature we all love to hear good things about us. There is a term current today called "positive stroking." It means saying good things to people about themselves to make them feel better.

True it is that we all need to hear encouraging, heartening words at times. But if we know our strong bent to be praised, to be "loved, honored, worshipped and adored," we should be leery of that within us that swells with pleasure when we are praised. "Well done!" is one thing, but being told we are wonderful is a different "kettle of fish."

How then do we receive rebuke from *anyone* if we believe we are wonderful? How could we? It would not seem fitting or proper or even truthful. Yet, as our Scripture tells us, "Surely there is not a righteous man on earth who does good and never sins" (v. 20). Somerset Maugham once observed, "People ask you for criticism, but they only want praise." That may be well and good for the world apart from God. It is not well and good for Christians who know "a more excellent way," the way of receiving correction and letting it work for us. "The rebuke of the wise" refers to something spoken out of greater light than we have at the moment, greater discernment and understanding. Most of us at times have such a word for others, and most of us have need of such a word from others. If we begin to see the love of God and the spirit of Jesus behind such words, then we can appreciate them for what they are.

> And blest is he who can divine
> Where the true right doth lie,
> And dares to take the side that seems
> Wrong to man's blindfold eye!
>
> Oh, learn to scorn the praise of men!
> Oh, learn to lose with God!
> For Jesus won the world through shame,
> And beckons thee his road.
>
> And right is right, since God is God;
> And right the day must win;
> To doubt would be disloyalty,
> To falter would be sin!
>
> *(Faber)*

1. What value do you think merciful honesty has in the 3D experience?

Do Not Be Weary of His Reproof

Daily Reading: Proverbs 3:1-12

My son, do not despise the Lord's discipline or be weary of His reproof, for the Lord reproves him whom He loves, as a father the son in whom he delights. (vv. 11,12)

Reproof and correction are expressions of love. These are the basic ideas of this entire week of 3D. It is vitally important that we learn the truth of this as we go on in our walk with Jesus Christ. The writer of the Proverbs encourages us to choose to see God's discipline and God's rebukes as expressions of His fatherly love and care for us.

Most of us are neophytes or newcomers to this concept. We may have accepted (even unwillingly) the fact that our parents did correct us in love, even though we know as parents ourselves, that parental correction does not always come without sin. Nevertheless, it is better for the child to be corrected than not to be corrected, and there are no sinless parents around, so we have to accept the fact that our parents did the best they knew, and be grateful for it. At the same time, we can commit ourselves as parents to do the best we know, and trust God with the results. It goes without saying that at the time, no discipline is welcomed by any child—but remembering back, we can testify that discipline did us good.

Even when we recognize the Lord's hand in a certain discipline, however, self-pity can still rise up and we can grow "weary of his reproof." Self-pity says, "It is too much. Even though I need to change or am wrong in such and such an area, this is unjust and too much!" Particularly if we have habitually comforted ourselves with food, drink, sleep, etc., we may be especially vulnerable at this point. This is when we need to gird up ourselves, call someone for help, get busy doing something to distract our self demands, and pray mightily for a new measure of grace and the presence of the Lord. Small victories lead to larger ones. Small indulgences lead to larger ones. The choice, in the midst of temptation, is ours.

A Prayer: *O God, Who hast folded back the mantle of the night to clothe us in the golden glory of the day, chase from our hearts all gloomy thoughts, and make us glad with the brightness of hope, that we may effectively aspire to unwon virtues, through Jesus Christ our Lord. Amen.* (Bp. Charles H. Brent)

1. Where this week have you seen reproof and correction are expressions of loving concern?

Week Review

This is something which is difficult to get across—and yet something we believe has changed many lives. In *Getting Your House in Order* there is a testimony about a woman who was challenged by another group member about not following her 3D disciplines. She was asked, "Why are you in this group? You never follow the diet, and you don't do the things we've all committed to do! . . ." That was a word of truth. As a result that very night she gave her life to Jesus Christ. Someone had loved her enough to correct her. That correction was a stepping stone for her into eternal life.

1. Did this topic sound a little stern when you began the week?

2. Did you feel more comfortable by the end of the week? Why?

3. Are you able to speak the truth in love to anyone around you?

4. Is anyone really honest with you?

SPIRITUAL JOURNAL

You need every pressure, every rejection, every sorrow and grief and blessing to bring you wholly to Jesus.

M. Cay & M. Judy

"If We Confess Our Sins"

"If we confess our sins, He is faithful and just, and will forgive our sins and cleanse us from all unrighteousness."

I John 1:9

I Know My Transgression

Daily Reading: Psalm 51

The fifty-first Psalm is perhaps the greatest prayer of confession ever composed. It came from the heart of one who was truly convicted of his sin, truly sorry for it, and who was willing to throw himself on the mercy of God in the belief that God is merciful to sinners. So it makes a good point at which to start this week's meditations on the combined subjects of "Repentance, Confession and Forgiveness."

The Holy Spirit is the spirit of truth. He searches out the inward parts, and reveals to us our condition. Thank God we have such an inward light. Jesus said, "If the light in you is darkness, how great is that darkness!" But we have the light of the Holy Spirit to shine like a floodlight on the sin areas, exposing all the hidden creepy-crawlies within.

We cannot repent when we do not know our transgression. It would be a terrible thing to be left in the darkness of delusion, because then we would be unable to repent. Like those people described in the first chapter of Romans, we would be "given up" by God to all that was within us. If you have ever had a good look at what is inside, you know that it is not very pretty to see. But when we have been convicted by the Holy Spirit of our transgression, we know our transgression, our wrongness, and we can then begin to repent. We can ask for mercy, for washing and cleansing, and like the Psalmist we can say to God, "thou art justified in thy sentence, and blameless in thy judgment." In other words, we agree with God's judgment about where we are wrong.

When a surgeon begins to operate on a person, he has to know where the trouble is—and have a pretty good idea what it is. And there is a lot about it that the patient would prefer to avoid, but knowing that what lies ahead is joy and health, goes through with the pain of it. That is a fairly accurate picture of the process of conviction and repentance. There is pain, and we might rather avoid it. But for the joy set before us, we endure it, knowing that in Jesus Christ there is mercy, forgiveness, restoration and joy!

A Prayer: *Come as the light; to us reveal*
Our emptiness and woe,
And lead us in those paths of life
Whereon the righteous go.

(Andrew Reed, 1829)

1. How did David react when confronted with his sin?

2. How do you respond when faced with your sin?

Week 8, Day 2

So Turn and Live

Daily Reading: Ezekiel 18:21-32

For I have no pleasure in the death of anyone, says the Lord God; so turn and live. (v. 32)

God is so loving, so giving, so generous that He desires to give life. He is the Source of life, and He created us for life. Throughout the Bible, we glean this picture of Him in His infinite patience with His people. He desires life for them all!

It is a reassuring and encouraging thought amid the struggles of our lives, to know that God desires life for us. Jesus said it in another way: "I have come that they may have life and have it abundantly." (John 10:10) It is not just existence that He gives us and desires for us. It is life in fullness and abundance, life as it was created to be in the heart of the Creator and that He longs to give His children.

What holds us back from that life? It can be nothing but ourselves. It cannot be that God is unable to give what He wills to give. No force in heaven or earth can stay His hand. But because of the unique place He has given us, He will not overrule or destroy our wills. He will not make robots out of us, even though He could. Instead, He allows us to stumble, to fall, to taste the fruit of our sin, to feel the pain of the separation we have made from Him—to the end that we will turn and live.

In this Ezekiel chapter, the wicked man is encouraged to turn from his way and live. The righteous man is encouraged not to turn from his way to die. God's will is life for us all. The way to life has been opened for us by our Lord Jesus Christ. He has fought the battle, and invites us to share in the benefits of His victory.

But in order to do that, we must turn, over and over again, when we have gone out of the way, when we have lapsed back into our old nature; then the way back is to turn from our way, to His way, and find that abundant life again. If you do not have a deep sense of repentance, pray for it. It is a precious gift which leads to life.

A Prayer Thought: *How true it is that if you fight with your conscience and lose, then you win.* *(J. Moulton Thomas)*

1. How is God's faithfulness demonstrated as we confess our sin?

No Longer Worthy

Daily Reading: Luke 15:11-32

This story of the prodigal son can be read with several different objects in mind—the merciful, waiting Father, the wayward but finally repentant son, or the jealous elder brother. Certainly one of its most endearing qualities, however, is its picture of a young man who decided to go his own way, found that all he thought would bring him happiness led him finally to being willing to eat pigs' food, and coming to his senses, returned to his father's house. What had happened inside that young man is the thing we need to see, as we think about repentance, confession and forgiveness.

First, his repentance came about when he realized where he was and what he had done. "He came to himself" (v. 17). We have talked about that in earlier devotional readings—this process of realizing who we are and what we have done. He no longer lived with blinders over his eyes, expecting that things would get better. He took responsibility for where he was, and decided to do something about it! "I will arise and go to my father!"

Second, his confession is expressed in these words: "Father, I have sinned against heaven and before you; I am no longer worthy to be called your son." Even though his father had come out to meet him "while he was yet at a distance," and had embraced and kissed him, the son knew what he had to say. He had to acknowledge with his words the reality of what he had seen about himself.

Third, his repentance and confession brought the assurance of forgiveness. They did not earn forgiveness, for you cannot earn forgiveness—it is a free gift. But they did enable him to receive and enjoy the father's forgiveness.

This is our pattern. It is God's pattern for us, and as we follow it, we enter over and over again into His fellowship as His beloved children.

> My God is reconciled;
> His pard'ning voice I hear;
> He owns me as His child;
> I can no longer fear.
> With confidence I now draw nigh,
> And, "Father, Abba, Father," cry!

(Charles Wesley)

1. How did the young man "come to himself"?

2. How do you take responsibility for "where you are" and decide to do something about it?

Confess Your Sins to One Another

Daily Reading: James 5

Therefore confess your sins to one another, and pray for one another that you may be healed. (v. 16)

When should we confess our sins to another person? That seems a legitimate question. Certainly it is unwise to confess sexual misconduct to anyone other than a trustworthy pastor, priest, or mature counselor. Otherwise, it can become a stumbling block and a snare. A timely warning against such an unwise course is in order!

There are, however, many sins which can and should be confessed to other Christians-to members of our group, prayer group, or wherever God has provided people willing to "bear one another's burdens, and so fulfill the law of Christ."

Sometimes confessing our sins in secret to God does not seem to bring relief from the burden or guilt of them, and we need additional help from others. Here again, Bonhoeffer's words seem appropriate:

God has willed that we should seek and find His living word in the witness of a brother, in the mouth of a man. Therefore, the Christian needs another Christian who speaks God's word to him. He needs him again and again when he becomes uncertain and discouraged, for by himself, he cannot help himself without belying the truth. He needs his brother man as a bearer and proclaimer of the divine word of salvation

That "word of salvation" is often the assurance of forgiveness after we have exposed our sin of jealousy, rebellion, hatred, or whatever. That we are loved and accepted, forgiven and cleansed is a cause of rejoicing and fellowship in the entire Body of Christ, represented by the small group in which we have made our confession.

That "word of salvation" may also be additional light thrown on the problem we are talking about, as we come to see more clearly that we are behaving out of subconscious, buried feelings and motivations. Once we see them, and they are brought into the light, we can have the peace of God which passes understanding. "And pray for one another, that you may be healed." The healing is first inward, and then, oftentimes physical as well.

> O Savior Christ, thou too art man;
> Thou has been troubled, tempted, tried;
> Thy kind but searching glance can scan
> The very wounds that shame would hide.   *(Henry Twells, 1868)*

1. When should we confess our sins to another person?

2. When recently have you received the assurance of forgiveness and experienced restored relationships after you've exposed and confessed your sin?

The Repentance of Nineveh

Daily Reading: Jonah 3

When God saw what they did, how they turned from their evil way, God repented of the evil which he had said he would do to them, and he did not do it. (v. 10)

Nineveh was renowned for its wickedness. In Chapter 1, God's word came to Jonah saying, "Arise, go to Nineveh, that great city, and cry against it; for their wickedness is come up before me." There was no doubt about Nineveh's need for repentance. But there is an unusual feature to this story. Apparently Jonah's message was only to "cry out" against Nineveh's sin and to declare its impending doom. There was no call for repentance as such. This should give us a clue as to how God sometimes deals with us. Something may come into our lives that seems clear-cut, definite, and unchangeable. It may be clear to us that it is the judgment of God on us, or someone may be angry with us for something we have done and cannot undo. What is our response? Anger? Self-defense? Hurt? Withdrawal and passivity?

A good example of what not to do in such a case is seen in I Samuel 3, where young Samuel was given a message to deliver to Eli, the priest, promising judgment on Eli's house because of his sons' wickedness. Eli's answer, "It is the Lord; let him do what seems good to him." (I Samuel 3:18) He made no effort to change!

But Nineveh was wiser in this case. Though the prophet did not hold out any hope, the king said, "Let us repent, and perhaps God will be gracious." And they did.

The implication here is that if the wicked people of Nineveh could repent, there is no reason that God's people cannot repent when confronted by the Holy Spirit with their wrongness. It is true today as it was then!

> Search out our hearts and make us true,
> Wishful to give to all their due;
> From love of pleasure, lure of gold
> From sins which make the heart grow cold
> Wean us and train us with thy rod;
> Teach us to know our faults, O God.
> *(William Boyd Carpenter, 1841-1918)*

1. If you are truly sorry for your sin, you will want to change. What specific steps are you taking to allow God to change you?

2. What is the difference between remorse and repentance?

Week 8, Day 6

Purified with Blood

Daily Reading: Hebrews 9

And without the shedding of blood there is no forgiveness of sins. (v. 22b)

The entire Old Testament sacrificial system begins to make sense when we see it as a foreshadowing of the "one, true, pure immortal sacrifice" of Jesus Christ. The blood of bulls and lambs and goats was shed in anticipation of the Lamb of God who would take away the sin of the world.

What does that mean to us as Christians? First, it means that the shedding of Jesus' Blood is a sacrifice for our sin, and that forgiveness and remission are applied when that sin is brought "under the blood." We need the soul-cleansing Blood to free us from the stain and pollution of sin. That comes about when we recognize the sin, take responsibility for it, confess it, and seek the Blood-washing. I John 1 says, "If we walk in the light, as He is in the light, we have fellowship with one another, and the blood of Jesus His Son cleanses us from all sin" (v. 7). Notice that it is when it is "in the light," and not hidden in the dark that we have the Blood-cleansing. I John 1 goes on to say, "If we say we have no sin, we deceive ourselves, and the truth is not in us." This clearly refers to our acknowledgement and confession of sin as a part of the cleansing and healing process.

Secondly, it says that our good works cannot make up for our wrongs. Too many of us fall back into the old pattern, even after becoming Christians, of trying to compensate for our wrongness by doing good or right things. The way out of sin is confession and forgiveness—not working harder at being right. Out of the blessedness of forgiveness, and the gratitude of our Lord for His sacrifice for us, we bring forth "works that befit repentance," the fruit of obedience in our lives.

But if we ever fall back into thinking that we do not need the shed Blood of Jesus, that our own goodness and righteousness is enough, then we have fallen from grace into dead works. No life comes forth from dead works, and we will be hardened Pharisees, while claiming with our lips our loyalty to Jesus. May God save us from such a fate!

1. Where have you seen this week that you've tried to make up for your wrongs by good works?

2. What does "the one true pure immortal sacrifice" of Jesus Christ mean to you personally?

He Will Forgive. . . and Cleanse

Daily Reading: I John 1

He is faithful and just, and will forgive us our sins, and cleanse us from all unrighteousness. (v. 9)

George Adam Smith wrote, "The forgiveness of God is the foundation of every bridge from a hopeless past to a courageous present."

That's what we need: a courageous present. A present that is as free from fears and hang-ups, from bondage to old habits and ways of reacting as is possible at this moment. We are not yet there, we are not yet perfect, we have not yet arrived-but we are on the way! Praise be to God!

"Why, then," you may ask, "all this talk about repentance and forgiveness? I'm a Christian, and Jesus forgave me my sins when I accepted Him, and He has cleansed me from the past!"

Indeed, as we came to Jesus in our need, He did forgive and cleanse. But we find that there are new expressions of the old self cropping up (or leaking out) all along the way. And we may get so discouraged that we might even wonder if we are Christians at all! That sad state has plagued many sincere people. They thought they had accepted Jesus with all their heart, but they did not find the ongoing victory they had heard about, and they felt that they either had to pretend to be better than they were, or find out why it was the way it was.

Here, in this little verse is the answer. What is born of God, the life of the Holy Spirit within us, does not sin. That is there, and it is given, the Presence of God within every true child of His.

But the old, Adamic nature is also there, seeking to express itself in the old patterns of hurt, desire to be loved, desire to be number one, to win, lusting after the things of this world. And there is the adversary, the Devil, using the old nature, appealing to it, and tempting us to wander far from the Lord. We all know the tug and pull of it.

But there is a way out of this mess. It begins here-"If we confess our sins, He is faithful and just, and will forgive us our sins and cleanse us from all unrighteousness." The more we learn it, believe it, and practice it, the more we can advance in our life in Christ.

1. What does it mean to you to be forgiven?

Week Review

We hope you've caught a glimpse from the Daily Devotional and the tape that it is safe to recognize and admit that we are sinners. We simply confess it, repent of it, receive forgiveness and go on in the joy of a soul set free, praying for the grace to change.

1. Do you believe that God sent His Son to die for wrong people, needy people, sinners and not those who consider themselves right? Why is that important to you?

2. Is it safe yet for you to be wrong?

3. Do you still think and feel that your acceptance by God, and by other people, is based on your goodness?

SPIRITUAL JOURNAL

The adamant "I am right" attitude is the basis of all division in the body of Christ.

M. Cay & M. Judy

Emotions: What to Do with Them

"Rejoice with those who rejoice, weep with those who weep."

Romans 12:15

The Anger and Sorrow of God

Daily Reading: Genesis 6:1-8, Deuteronomy 9:13-29

And the Lord was sorry that he had made man on earth, and it grieved him in his heart. (Gen. 6:6) And the Lord was so angry with Aaron that he was ready to destroy him. (Deut. 9:20)

These and many other passages show us what we could term the "emotions of God." The Bible does not reveal a God who is placid, without feeling, dwelling in eternal calm. It reveals to us a God who acts, speaks, and yes, feels.

What are some of the things that bring sorrow to God? "Woe to those," says the prophet Amos, "who lie on beds of ivory, and stretch themselves on their couches, eat lambs from the flock . . . sing idle songs . . . drink wine in bowls, and anoint themselves with the finest oils, but are not grieved over the ruin of Joseph!" (Amos 6:4—6) The ruin of His people, the sin that blemishes and deforms His creation—these bring grief and sorrow to the Father's heart.

What produces anger? In the Scripture for today, it is clear that the readiness of the people to trample underfoot all that God had done for them, the miracles of the Passover, the Red Sea, and all the other deliverances—and to turn away to their own inventions—this kindled the holy anger, the righteous wrath of a Holy God.

This week we are looking at emotions, and asking what we can and should do about them. It is good in the beginning to see that some of the emotions we least want to recognize in ourselves are attributed to God Himself in the Bible. His, of course, are without sin. Ours are not. But knowing that God, too, feels anger, grief, sorrow, and the like, should make it easier to see that it is all right to recognize these in ourselves. Pray this week that the Lord will give you grace to get in touch with your real feelings and begin to learn how to deal with them more constructively.

A Prayer Thought: *There is no place where earth's sorrows are more felt than up in heaven; there is no place where earth's failings have such kindly judgment given.* *(F. W. Faber, 1814-1863)*

1. What does it mean to you to know that God feels all your sorrows and griefs?

2. Is it a relief to you to consider that it is safe to recognize feelings that you have such as anger, jealousy, and fear? Why?

The Rejoicing of God

Daily Reading: Isaiah 62

As the bridegroom rejoices over the bride, so shall your God rejoice over you. (v. 5)

As we think about our emotions, it is good to see how the Bible also ascribes emotions or feelings to God. Here is a good example of God being pictured as rejoicing over His people. In Luke 15, Jesus reminds us that there is great rejoicing in heaven over one sinner who repents.

All of this should help us to see that our feelings are an integral and essential part of being made in the image of God. Because we *can* feel joy, love, sorrow, grief, anger, and so on, we are *persons*.

If we do not deal with our negative emotions, it is a sad truth that we lose the ability to rejoice. The entire feeling level becomes so depressed or repressed that it becomes impossible for us to experience the excitement and joy we may have known as children. No wonder Jesus said, "Except you are converted and become as little children, you cannot enter the kingdom of God" (Matt. 18:3). We need to treasure and, if necessary, recapture our ability to truly rejoice. Only then can we be in harmony with heaven which rejoices over one sinner who repents, and with God, who rejoices as a bridegroom rejoices over his bride.

Couple this with such commands to us as these: "Rejoice always" (I Thessalonians 5:16), "Rejoice in the Lord always; again I will say, Rejoice" (Philippians 4:4).

The ability to rejoice is commensurate with our wholeness in the Lord. Never take it for granted, or think that it is all right if you grow dull in your willingness to rejoice!

> Let all the world in every corner sing,
> My God and King!
> The heavens are not too high,
> His praise may thither fly;
> The earth is not too low,
> His praises there may grow.
> Let all the world in every corner sing,
> My God and King!
>
> *(George Herbert, 1633)*

1. Where have you seen that when you refuse to deal with your negative emotions you lose the ability to rejoice?

A Man of Sorrows

Daily Reading: John 11:1-44

When Jesus saw her weeping, and the Jews who came with her also weeping, he was deeply moved in spirit and troubled; and he said, "Where have you laid him?" They said to him, "Lord, come and see." Jesus wept. (vv. 33-35)

The prophet Isaiah called him "a man of sorrows and acquainted with grief."

"Is it for nothing," asks one, "that the Evangelist, some sixty years after it occurred, holds up to all ages with such touching brevity the sublime spectacle of *the Son of God in tears?* What a seal of His perfect oneness with us in the most redeeming feature of our stricken humanity . . . The tears of Mary and her friends acted sympathetically upon Him, and drew forth His emotions. What a vivid outcoming of real humanity!"

Knowing that we have a great High Priest who is able "to sympathize with our weaknesses" (Heb. 4:15), we should not be ashamed to face our own feelings of weakness, sorrow, grief, fear and need. These things we often try to deny, but it is very encouraging to know that Jesus did not try to hide them. He was indeed an example to us, the example of perfect manhood. But we have thought that such feelings were unacceptable, and many of us have made a practice of denying them—so that we become deadened inside and may not know how we feel on any given subject, because we do not feel anything very much. Such a state is unnecessary for a Christian to remain in, and we can begin to get in touch with feelings—good, bad, and in between. The more we allow our feelings to surface, the freer we become to grow into the kind of whole people we were meant to be.

A Prayer: *Lord Jesus, we read that in the days of Your flesh, You offered up prayers and supplications with loud cries and tears (Heb. 5:7). May I not be ashamed to cry when I need to, and laugh when it is fitting, and become the whole person You want me to be. In Your Name. Amen.*

1. What unacceptable feelings have you sought to deny?

2. How do you express positive emotions? Negative emotions?

Be Angry and Sin Not

Daily Reading: Ephesians 4:17-32

Be angry but do not sin; do not let the sun go down on your anger. (v. 26)

Charles Haddon Spurgeon, the great English 19th-century preacher, has an interesting word to say about anger:

"Anger is not always or necessarily sinful, but it has such a tendency to run wild that whenever it displays itself we should be quick to question its character with this enquiry: 'Doest thou well to be angry?' It may be that we can answer, 'Yes.' Very frequently anger is the madman's firebrand, but sometimes it is Elijah's fire from heaven. We do well when we are angry with sin because of the wrong it commits against our good and gracious God, or with ourselves because we remain so foolish after so much divine instruction, or with others when the sole cause of anger is the evil they do. He who is not angry at transgression becomes a partaker in it. Sin is a loathsome and hateful thing, and no renewed heart can patiently endure it. God Himself is angry with the wicked every day, and it is written in His Word, 'Ye that love the Lord, hate evil.' "

The Apostle here seems to differentiate between being angry and sinning. Yet many of us have been so conditioned to think of anger as always being wrong and ugly, and we have so wanted not to be wrong and ugly, that we have repressed the anger that came up in us, and tried to deny its very existence! It may even have been "righteous anger," a justifiable reaction to sin and the harm that it was causing in someone else's life. But if we think that anger is not becoming to a Christian, that we are always supposed to be calm and unflappable, then our tendency will be to push it down and deny its existence.

Here the Bible is saying, "Be angry, but do not sin." Phillips translates it like this: "If you are angry, be sure that it is not a sinful anger. Never go to bed angry— don't give the devil that sort of foothold!" When we check out our anger and find that it is sinful and wrong, we should be quick to do something about it. On the other hand, we must allow room for the fact that being who we are, we do get angry, and that it is a part of our essential emotional make-up that we can get angry. Many of us need much freeing of bottled-up anger which we have not admitted to ourselves.

1. List the things that make you angry.

2. What do you do with your anger?—confess it, push it down inside you, or refuse to recognize it?

When I Am Afraid

Daily Reading: Psalm 55,56

When I am afraid, I put my trust in thee. (Psalm 56, v.3)

Fear is one of the "basic emotions" with which we are made. It has a very important function in our lives, warning us of danger, enabling us to put forth greater effort when needed, and so on. A healthy fear is essential to our well-being.

Moreover, we are told, "The fear of the Lord is the beginning of wisdom." We need to have a holy fear of God—knowing that He is our Maker and we are accountable to Him. Without it, it is doubtful that we will be moved toward obedience. Few if any of us could claim to obey solely on the basis of our love for God.

Yet, "perfect love casts out fear." There is in fear the potentiality of going beyond its useful function, and becoming a devastating and controlling emotion. Fear then becomes the enemy. ("We have nothing to fear but fear itself," said a famous President once.) Satan uses fear to paralyze, to make us hesitant when we should be bold, and to sap our energy and distract our attention from the Lord.

The Psalmist knew what it was to be afraid. In Psalm 55:4,5 he says, "The terrors of death have fallen upon me. Fear and trembling come upon me, and sorrow overwhelms me." Fear, when it reaches such proportions can cause tragic results.

So what is the solution? First, not to deny its reality. One of the most dangerous and foolish things is to "pretend to be brave" when we are not! Fear cannot be controlled in that way. Rather, we need to face its presence and *confess* it to the Lord. "When I am afraid." Not if, but *when.* We all are at times, when our lives seem out of control: at news of an accident, or illness or when we are informed that we ourselves may be in danger of some unknown illness. Confess to the Lord that you are afraid, and that it is because you do not trust Him as you should! He is trustworthy! That's what the Psalmist is saying. God "whose word I praise, in God I trust without a fear." We can move from fear to faith—over and over again, because we can *choose* to trust in our Heavenly Father!

A Prayer: I call upon You, Lord, and You will save me. I utter my complaints and my moans, and You hear my voice. What then can flesh do to me? By grace, I choose to give up my fear and trust you more and more. In Jesus' Name. Amen.

1. List the fears in your life.

2. How can you move from fear to faith over and over again?

Learning to be Genuine

Daily Reading: Romans 12

Let love be genuine; hate what is evil; hold fast to what is good; love one another with brotherly affection; outdo one another in showing honor. (vv. 9, 10)

This week we are talking about what to do with our emotions, with a lot of emphasis on facing them as a real part of our lives. Hiding them, denying them, disowning them, if you will, are the most harmful ways of dealing with them.

The goal of the Christian life is to become integrated, whole persons, God-directed instead of self-directed. The wholeness comes as we are inwardly healed by the presence of the Holy Spirit, enlightened by the truth. In another way of describing it, we might say that it means having all our parts connected correctly to one another and functioning as God created them to function.

This twelfth chapter of Romans deals with our relationships with one another in the Christian fellowship. The Apostle recognizes that there are forces outside and inside that keep us from being what Jesus Christ means us to be. "Do not be conformed to this world" (v. 2). The world is constantly trying to "press us into its mold," as someone has put it. And we must resist by allowing the transforming power of God to work in us. But there are inner forces, too, which distort us— "I bid every one among you not to think of himself more highly than he ought to think" (v. 3). Can we plead innocent on that one? Thinking too highly of ourselves opens us up to get hurt, feel rejected, to become jealous, and, in general, to infuse a dark, negative element into the Christian fellowship. What can we do about it? Unfortunately, what some people do, is to try to cover it up with a surface politeness and friendliness, which belies what is underneath. So Paul says, "Let love be genuine." Let it be sincere. But we cannot be sincere unless we honestly deal with the negative feelings we have about one another. *Then,* by God's grace, love does flow through us to others, and we can receive God's love through them to us. Love becomes genuine as we become real, because of Jesus Christ.

A Prayer: *Lord, let me learn to be real, that my love may become genuine. In Jesus' Name. Amen.*

We cannot be sincere and have genuine love unless we deal with the negative feelings we have towards one another.

1. What negative feelings do you have towards people you live with, your friends, and the group?

2. What can you do with these negative feelings?

First the Inside

Daily Reading: Matthew 23:1-28

Woe to you, scribes and Pharisees, hypocrites! for you cleanse the outside of the cup and of the plate, but inside they are full of extortion and rapacity. You blind Pharisees! First cleanse the inside of the cup and of the plate, that the outside also may be clean. (vv. 25,26)

The scribes and Pharisees were caught up in outward performance and appearance. They did not set out to be hypocrites; they just *were* hypocrites because they had been blinded by their own rightness.

Jesus did not encourage "bad behavior." But neither was he put off by "good behavior." He looked beyond the outward pattern to see what was in the heart. And in the hearts of the Pharisees, he saw self-deception and hypocrisy.

We need to take this to ourselves. When we have made a life-pattern of denying feelings we had-ugly, wrong feelings that needed to be dealt with-we can be nothing but hypocrites. It is not that we mean to be hypocrites; we just are, because we are not connected up right. Our feelings and our ideas are not "tracking together," as the phrase goes.

Even when our words and our faces express joy or love, or some other positive emotion, if our heart is not right, then what comes out of us is cloudy, confusing, and hurtful. There is no way around it: either we have to learn to be honest with ourselves and others, or we will continue to live in the same darkness that the Pharisees lived in. They could not hear what Jesus was saying, because their hearts kept telling them he was wrong and they were right.

Facing our ugly emotions, admitting them before the Lord and one another, and seeking His power in overcoming them, is the healthy wholesome Way into fuller, freer life. The Pharisees, for the most part, stayed in their sin of delusion. We do not have to, for we know Jesus Christ has the answer to our needs.

A Prayer: *Thank You, Lord, that I do not have to deny my negative feelings nor live in them. There is a way out, through You. Thank You that You love me so much that You are leading me, day by day, in finding that way. Amen.*

1. This week what ugly emotions have you faced? Have you admitted them before the Lord and one another?

2. How are you seeking His power to overcome them?

Week Review

Emotions help us express what is going on inside of us, and we do not need to be afraid of them. While on the diet you have been happy when you have lost weight, and then you have been unhappy when you did not lose any. Also, it is often our emotions that cause us to overeat or undereat. As you begin to recognize these emotions, positive or negative, and ask the Lord to help you to not be controlled by them, your eating and whole life can come into balance.

1. What emotions are you most aware of in your life?

2. Have you seen any relationship between your emotions and your eating habits?

3. Are there any feelings that you try to hide from yourself or others?

4. What does God want us to do with our emotions?

SPIRITUAL JOURNAL

As you build patterns of obedience your emotions begin to change.

M. Cay & M. Judy

When Light is Darkness

"You will know the truth, and the truth will make you free."

John 8:32

The Truth Will Make You Free

Daily Reading: John 8:31-59

If you continue in My word, you are truly My disciples, and you will know the truth, and the truth will make you free. (vv. 31, 32)

This week we are thinking about the "lies we believe." By that we mean that many things we have been taught, or have picked up ourselves, which we have believed to be true, are in reality *false*.

Perhaps you have never thought much about it. But think a moment. If you think something is true, and act upon it, it makes a great deal of difference whether it is true or not.

There was a story told years ago about a worker in a factory whose clothing caught fire. A fellow worker grabbed a bucket labeled "water," (as factories had in those days) and threw it on his co-worker. But the bucket contained gasoline. It was labeled wrong!

Think about that in connection with things we believe to be true, some of which are mentioned in your Bible Studies this week. How vital it is for your own welfare and that of others, to begin to be able to discern truth from falsehood.

Jesus said, "If you continue in My word. . . ." That is a clue. He not only has the truth, He is the Truth, and we can expect His active help and assistance as we seek to come more and more into the truth that sets free.

This week should be an exciting one, as you begin to discover lies which you have thought to be truth, and start on the adventure of renouncing the lies (for Satan is the father of lies) and affirming the truth (for Jesus is the Truth).

Expect miracles!

1. Can you think of one "truth" in your life that turned out later to be a lie?

2. How has believing that lie affected your life?

If the Light in You Is Darkness

Daily Reading: Matthew 6

But if your eye is not sound, your whole body will be full of darkness. If then the light in you is darkness, how great is the darkness! (v. 23)

Throughout history, further light has proved old light to be darkness. For many centuries theories about the universe, about the human body, about the shape and structure of the earth prevailed. Then discoveries proved old theories wrong and made new advances possible. Perhaps nowhere has this been more dramatic than in the advance of medical science.

A poet said it like this:

> New occasions teach new duties,
> Time makes ancient good uncouth.
> They must upward still and onward
> Who would keep abreast of truth.

(James Russell Lowell)

Because we live by faith rather than facts provable in a laboratory, it is possible to think that "one opinion is as good as another." But Jesus issues a stern warning against such a relativity. He plainly says that unless what comes in is real light, then what we think is light is really darkness. The Old Testament is the history of the struggle of Truth, the Truth about God and His Nature and His Purposes, against the false gods of the nations. If we Christians are to be the light of the world, as Jesus said we are, then we must be careful to reject false ideas, especially our own false ideas about ourselves and what makes life enjoyable, and "buy the truth and sell it not!" (Proverbs 23:23)

Keep at it, and seek the Spirit of Truth to show up the many wrong things you believe about what makes life worth living. You may be surprised how many they are!

A Prayer: *Spirit of Truth, prevail! In Jesus' Name. Amen.*

1. Do you believe that correction is rejection? Why?

2. How would your life be different if you knew that correction is not rejection but really love?

Recognizing and Destroying Delusion

Daily Reading: Acts 19:1-20

And a number of those who practiced magic arts brought their books together and burned them in the sight of all; and they counted the value of them and found it came to fifty thousand pieces of silver. So the word of the Lord grew and prevailed mightily. (vv. 19,20)

The whole area around Ephesus was shaken and affected by the gospel. God's power was evidenced in the changed lives and the healings, both physical and emotional, which accompanied the preaching of Paul.

Satan sought to frustrate and hinder the work, but God's word prevailed over all opposition. The influence which the Truth had is clearly seen in this passage, as we read the summary of the two years' work of Paul in Ephesus. Those who had become believers "came, confessing and divulging their practices" (v. 18). The Lord was putting the power of the Truth alongside the power of the evil lies by which these people had lived, and they came to see that, whereas lies bind and delude, the Truth frees. So they brought out this horde of books on magical arts and occult practices, knowing that they had been in bondage to the prince of lies, Satan himself!

The delusions by which Satan seeks to bind us are based on our human sinful desire to be God. Since this is the same nature he, Satan, has, he recognizes its likeness in our fallen nature, and appeals to it. His lies offer us instant gratification, pleasure without pain, without responsibility, and without price. But one does not go very far down that path without seeing that something is wrong. Still, we may go on in delusions of various kinds for many years, because they appeal to our vanity and ego and desire for an easy way.

How wonderful it is that when we taste the Truth, and get a foretaste of what it means to be a child of God, that we begin to get willing to pay the price of going further into the Truth. These people brought their books, which represented an investment that is staggering to the imagination even by today's standards. It was a price to pay-but they paid it gladly, for they were beginning to taste what it really means to be free. So the word of the Lord grew and prevailed mightily. May it grow and prevail mightily in us, too. Amen!

1. A few lies you may believe and live by:
    -Peace at any price is good.
    -Being hurt is the worst thing in the world.
    -If you love me you'll accept me as I am.
   Are you willing to see these as lies and choose truth?

2. What would be the truth instead of these?

How Long will You Seek After Lies

Daily Reading: Psalms 4,5

O Men, how long shall my honor suffer shame? How long will you love vain words and seek after lies? (Psalm 4:2)

We are told that the Hebrew word in this verse of "O men" is a word denoting distinction and honor. "God ironically gives them this title of honor in reference to their own high opinion of themselves."

These Psalms seem originally to refer to those who had joined David's son Absalom in rebellion against their anointed king. "How long will you seek after lies?" he asks, because they deluded themselves as to what was really going on. Absalom had used religion to cloak his real purpose (II Samuel 15:7,8) and had relied on falsehood and flattery to draw the people to himself and away from his father. Thus the entire project would collapse because it was based on lies and treason.

Why do we "seek after lies"? Is it not because, like these "distinguished men of honor," we prefer them to the hard truth? Do we not rather seek those who tell us good things about us, and tend to avoid those who tell us "bad things"?

We can see a parallel between them and ourselves-as long as we avoid the truth.

A Prayer: *May Your Spirit, O Lord, Who proceeds from You, illuminate our minds, and as Your Son promised, lead us into all truth, through the same Your Son Jesus Christ our Lord. Amen.*

1. Ask God to reveal specific lies you have believed that have controlled and influenced your life. List.

Misplaced Trust

Daily Reading: Jeremiah 7:1-20

Behold, you trust in deceptive words to no avail. (v. 8)

Judah thought that since they had the Temple of the Lord in their midst, and since they were God's chosen people, all would surely be well. The prophet is warning them that it makes no difference how much they trust "deceptive words"— it will do them no good. God holds them accountable for their faithfulness or lack of it to Himself, and all their wishful thinking will not stay His judgment. He reminds them that they can go to Shiloh, once the mighty capital of Israel after the kingdoms had divided in two following the death of Solomon. Shiloh was a great city, full of wealth and military power, proud and lifted up. But when Jeremiah spoke, the people were reminded that Shiloh was only a memory. "Go and see for yourself," they were told.

It was a stern lesson, but coupled with the positive side of our weekly theme, it is vitally important. Our trust will betray us if it is misplaced. If we build our lives and hopes on lies and delusions, they will not, cannot save us.

Instead, the truth is offered each one of us as we are open to it. We know the folly of some of the delusions we have entertained. There are more-for all of us. And God will lead you step by step in discovering and discarding them.

When you find that you have been believing a lie, pray something like this: "Lord, I confess that I have believed a lie. (State what it is.) I take responsibility for believing this, and I am sorry for it. I accept your forgiveness. I renounce this lie and all its effects in my life. I state the truth. (State the truth which you have seen in the place where you believed the lie.) I ask you to fill me with this truth, and let it bear fruit in my life. In Jesus' Name." Do this with each false idea and each delusion you discover you have believed. The effect is truly remarkable.

1. Why is truth so important for us from God's point of view?

Obeying the Truth

Daily Reading: Galatians 5:1-25

You were running well; who hindered you from obeying the truth? (v. 7)

The Galatian Christians were young in the faith. They had heard Paul's preaching about Jesus, and they had believed what he said, and they had accepted Jesus Christ as their Lord and Savior. The Holy Spirit was a reality in their lives, and they found their lives totally different from the old days.

But they were not stable, mature people. They quickly turned to listen to others who came telling about Jesus, who convinced them that in addition to believing, they also had to be circumcised and keep the Jewish law. They were persuaded that they would be superior Christians if they followed this new plan.

Paul was furious with those who had come and unsettled his converts. He had risked his life over and over again to carry the Good News to those who had not heard it. And now the Judaizers had slipped in behind him and were sowing confusion and controversy in the Church. The Letter to the Galatians could be called a "correction" letter, because Paul in his love and concern for them fears that they are going to turn to "another gospel," and turn away from the truth.

"You were running well," he says; "who hindered you from obeying the truth?" Probably the biggest thing that had hindered them was their desire to be right. This is in many ways the deadliest foe for Christians, because it is a counterfeit for being obedient. On the one hand, we are called to be obedient, but on the other, being right has subtle pride built in it that robs God of His glory and feeds our self-righteous, high opinion of ourselves. This is one of the hardest but most important lessons Christians have to learn. The truth makes us free to "walk in the Spirit," not gratifying the demands of the flesh, which includes "self-conceit" and "envy," as well as the gross sins of the flesh. One could well spend some time in prayer asking that the Spirit of Truth reveal where we are striving to be right instead of striving to be obedient.

Unless we obey the truth, we will fall prey to the subtle lies of the enemy. Truth is not only to be believed. It is to be obeyed.

A Prayer: *Lord Jesus, I see Your obedience to the truth, to Your Father's will. As You show me the truth, help me to treasure it and to obey it, so that I neither fall into sin nor run into any kind of danger. Amen.*

1. Truth is not only to be believed. It is to be obeyed. In your life, where do you see the truth that you should obey?

I Would Have Been Untrue

Daily Reading: Psalm 73

If I had said, "I will speak thus," I would have been untrue to the generation of thy children. (v. 15)

The Psalmist believed alot of things that were untrue. He looked about him, and saw arrogant, wicked men prospering. They seemed to have healthier bodies, less trouble, more success than people who were striving to do right. He looked at their pride and their violence. "Their eyes swell out with fatness, their hearts overflow with follies." They were contemptuous of others, and even snickered their blasphemies against God.

Then he noticed something else. In spite of all this (or because of it!) they were praised as though they had no faults!

Bitterness entered his heart. "It's no use trying to serve God and keep one's hands innocent of wrong," he thought.

But wait—"If I had said, 'I will speak thus,' I would have been untrue to the generation of thy children." Something stopped him when he went into the House of God. There he saw a deeper truth, and he knew that if he had allowed the jealous, envious feelings and thoughts about the wicked to stay in his heart, he would have betrayed others as well as himself.

When we harbor lies and delusions in our hearts, we are a menace to others as well as ourselves. For what comes out of our mouths will be accusing words against God, words which can mislead and cause others to stumble. And we all have been guilty of this.

"When my soul was embittered. . . I was stupid and ignorant!" says the Psalmist. And when we allow ourselves to become full of bitterness, we are just the same!

"Truly God is good to the upright!" (v. 1) "But for me, it is good to be near God" (v. 28). That is a place reserved for those who seek Him. The Father's presence is for those who love Him. Let the wicked and arrogant go. God is our strength and portion forever!

A Prayer: *When I am tempted to envy the godless, turn my eyes away to Thee, Lord Jesus. Thou art my joy, my hope, and my life. May that truth steady me to the end. Amen.*

1. What else has God shown you this week about living in truth versus living in falsehood?

Week Review

We have considered this week that many things we believe and have based our lives on, which we have believed to be true, are in reality, false.

1. What difference do you think believing and living by the truth should make in your life?

2. Does the word "lie" seem so ugly and "sinful" to you that you find it hard to consider there might be lies in your own life? Why?

3. What about "little white lies"? Do you ever tell them? Give some examples.

SPIRITUAL JOURNAL

The easiest way to get into trouble is to tell a tiny lie, believe a tiny lie, and leave out a tiny bit of truth.

M. Cay & M. Judy

Your Mind: A Battleground

"We destroy arguments and every proud obstacle to the knowledge of God, and take every thought captive to obey Christ."

II Corinthians 10:5

We Destroy Arguments

Daily Reading: II Corinthians 10

We destroy arguments and every proud obstacle to the knowledge of God, and taken every thought captive to obey Christ. (v. 5)

This week we are thinking together about the battle which goes on in our minds—the battle between light and darkness, between the Lord and the devil, between the Spirit and the flesh. It *is* the battleground on which the Christian's primary warfare is to be fought.

Paul is writing to the Corinthians, a particularly arrogant and haughty group of Christians. He knows that they listen to "arguments," because they allow their minds to become captivated with the wrong kind of thinking. How often do we indulge in imaginary conversations in our minds, thinking of the clever things we might have said, if only we had thought of them in time? We may be thinking of things we hope to say when we have the opportunity. Perhaps our thoughts may grow out of anxiety and fear, as we try to figure out a way to prevent some fearful thing from happening. At any rate, these vain imaginations are a part of the weaponry of our adversary, the devil, and if we do not recognize him, then we fall headlong into his trap.

"We destroy arguments," says St Paul. How? *By the truth.* Martin Luther's great hymn says it thus:

And though this world, with devils filled
Should threaten to undo us,
We will not fear, for God has willed
His truth to triumph through us.

The prince of darkness grim,
We tremble not for him;
His rage we can endure,
For lo! his doom is sure:
One little word shall fell him.

Satan's deceptive arguments are destroyed when we begin to recognize them for what they are, and apply the light of truth against them. In the name and power of Jesus Christ, we can win the battle!

A Prayer: *O Lord of Hosts! Enable us to fight the good fight of faith; to recognize the wiles of the enemy, and to bring every thought captive to obey Christ. We ask it in His Name, Amen.*

1. Be perfectly honest and write down some of the thoughts that run through your mind in a single day.

2. Make a list of the thoughts that are good constructive thoughts.

3. Make another list of bad thoughts—thoughts of jealousy, anger, lust, fantasy or day dreaming.

The Case of Judas

Daily Reading: Luke 22:1-33

Then Satan entered into Judas called Iscariot, who was of the number of the twelve; he went away and conferred with the chief priest and captains, how he might betray him to them. (vv. 3, 4)

Judas has been the subject of many studies. What made him do as he did! Surely he did not join the disciples with the idea of becoming the betrayer. Nothing in the Gospels indicates that he did. In John's Gospel we do read "he was a thief, and as he had the money box he used to take what was in it" (John 12:6b). In other words, he pilfered from the funds of the group for his own purposes, and thought it was hidden from the others. What does this suggest to you? That it is dangerous to try to get away with little things—little dishonesties, little "harmless" lies. This may be especially tempting in the food department when we are on some kind of special discipline. Are you absolutely honest in filling out your food sheets?

The danger with these little dishonesties is that they open up our minds to Satan's further plans. Do you remember the "Cat in the Hat" stories of Dr. Seuss? When the children opened the door to the "Cat in the Hat," he, the cat, took over from there on, and they watched in amazement and consternation at his antics. That, it seems, is a humorous picture of what happens when we inadvertently let Satan in through some "harmless" dishonesty. His plans are for your destruction, gradually or quickly. The battle becomes joined when you or I give him ground through our sin, for he has a right to any area where we have given him permission to come in. We give this permission by entering into sin. His reasonings may sound perfectly harmless and logical. But they are leading us into harmful paths. That is why the Lord taught us to pre-pray against temptation, and for Divine protection. We do not always recognize it when it comes! This is the subtlety of the battle for the mind, for we can be in the thick of it and not even know it is going on.

Judas stands as an extreme and tragic example of one whose "little sins" led him progressively into greater darkness. Instead of thinking of Judas as different from ourselves, we should recognize the same potentiality in ourselves of being deluded and becoming betrayers of the very One we seek to follow.

A Prayer: *Stab me awake, Lord, to the danger of letting my thoughts run into paths of jealousy, resentment, lust and vindictiveness. Help me not to give the enemy ground to destroy Your work in me. In Jesus' Name. Amen.*

1. Are you able to control your thoughts, or do your thoughts control you?

2. What are your most difficult thoughts to deal with?

Out of the Abundance of the Heart

Daily Reading: Luke 6:17-49

The good man out of the good treasure of his heart produces good, and the evil man out of his evil treasure produces evil; for out of the abundance of the heart his mouth speaks. (v. 45)

God knows and Satan knows that it is in the "heart," (read "mind") that our actions flow. Some of them come out of our subconscious, and we do not even understand what we are doing. Paul talks about this dilemma in Romans 7. But there is the need to do battle against the "evil" thoughts which seek to invade our minds at a conscious level. Then the Holy Spirit will bring to light those things that are buried in the unconscious which we need to be aware of, so that we do not have to fear them or be controlled by them.

What happens when a dark, evil thought enters your mind? Do you greet it, welcome it, entertain it, and hold friendly discourse with it? Do you assume that it is correct in all its suspicions, in its judgments against your fellow men, in its dark and jealous feelings of resentments that others have what you would like to have? If so, you are storing up a horde of "evil treasure," and out of that abundance your mouth will speak.

Do you ever surprise yourself by making some cutting remark (perhaps humorously disguised) that really puts another person "in his place"? If so, it may be because you have stored up a treasure of evil thoughts and feelings against him.

What can be done to rid ourselves of the horde of evil treasure (we all have some of them, of course), and to build up for ourselves a store of "good treasure" so that our words and actions can be consistent with our Christian commitment!

First, you can do battle with these thoughts when they come. Confess your jealousy, your resentment, your greed—or whatever—to the Lord as soon as the thoughts begin to appear. Then tell Satan to go with his thoughts in the Name of Jesus, and begin to pray positively for the person against whom you have harbored hurt, etc. It does work! And you can begin to see and tell the difference. Try it today!

A Prayer: *Arm me for battle, Lord, against all the wiles of the devil. Help me to be watchful and alert and ready to guard that which is good, which comes from You. I reject everything from Satan, and I choose everything from Jesus Christ. Amen.*

1. Is there anyone about whom you particularly think bad thoughts? Who? Why?

2. When is the best time to attack and do battle with a thought?

Blinded Minds

Daily Reading: II Corinthians 4

In their case the god of this world has blinded the minds of the unbelievers, to keep them from seeing the light of the gospel of the glory of Christ, who is the likeness of God. (v. 4)

All this week we are thinking about light and darkness in our minds, and the struggle between the two that is going on. Paul here clearly describes the unbelieving world as being "blinded" by the god of this world, Satan. In Chapter 3, he speaks of Israel's mind as being "hardened" (v. 14), so that when they read the Old Testament, their eyes are veiled and they do not perceive the truth they are reading. There is a relationship between the "hardening" and the "blindness" being spoken of here.

When we harden our minds to the truth of God, our minds become progressively darkened. Eventually we cannot discern truth from falsehood, and we are then in total deception about reality. You can see this in people who have become increasingly unreachable by others until they finally are hospitalized "out of reality." It is not mysterious; it is a process by which the mind hardened against seeing its wrongness becomes more and more right and unreachable, until it is completely "blind."

"This happened in the case of Tom, a splendid young man in his early twenties. Tom had tried for days to argue with me on the hate-filled issues of neo-Nazism, anti-Semitism, and white racism. Finally I turned to Tom and asked, 'Which do you want—to be right on these issues or to get well so as to leave this hospital!'

"Without a moment's hesitation he answered, 'Be right! I don't care if I never get out of this hospital!' " (Kingdom of Self, Earl Jabay, p. 27)

Let us pray for a new awareness of those things which harden our hearts and blind our minds, so that our minds may be filled with God's light and truth, and so that His wholeness may be manifest in us.

A Prayer: Lord, let it be so, In Jesus' Name. Amen.

1. What is the best way of dealing with evil thoughts?

2. What part do work and/or disciplines play in this battle?

Week 11, Day 5

The Wiles of the Devil

Daily Reading: Ephesians 6

Put on the whole armor of God, that you may be able to stand against the wiles of the devil. (v. 11)

According to the dictionary, a *wile* is "a trick or stratagem intended to ensnare or deceive." It is certainly possible to become too "devil-conscious," and to have an unhealthy attention to what we think are evidences of his presence or power. But it is equally possible to be so unaware of his wiles that we become easily ensnared by them, without ever knowing what is happening. Paul here is cautioning us to recognize that there are spiritual enemies arrayed against us. "We are not contending against flesh and blood, but against the principalities, against the powers, against the world rulers of this present darkness, against the spiritual hosts of wickedness in the heavenly places" (v. 12). These are all unseen forces or powers at work against us, and if we are not aware of them, how can we fight against them?

What are some of the "wiles of the devil," the tricks by which we are readily ensnared or deceived? Some of them may be;

. . . we are tempted to think too highly of ourselves or something we have done, making us overly sensitive to criticism or lack of praise.

. . . we may suddenly find ourselves very suspicious of others, and looking for ways to be hurt by them.

. . . we are tempted to think that we are hopeless, or our situation is hopeless.

. . . we are tempted to think that no one understands us, and that eating, or drinking, or whatever it is we want to do will not make any difference to anyone else.

Perhaps you may know how the tricks work in your own case. The mind is the battleground in which these tricks or wiles must be fought. If we accept lies as the truth, then we are on slippery ground indeed! The whole armor of God is needed and is available to us, when we recognize our need of His help.

1. How do you think we should try to fight against mind wandering and encourage spiritually healthy thoughts?

The Renewal of Your Minds

Daily Reading: Romans 12

Do not be conformed to this world, but be transformed by the renewal of your mind, that you may prove what is the will of God, what is good and acceptable and perfect. (v. 2)

> Dear Lord and Father of mankind
> Forgive our foolish ways.
> Reclothe us in our rightful minds,
> In purer lives thy service find,
> In deeper reverence, praise.
>
> *(Whittier)*

Our minds need to be "renewed." They were darkened by the fall of our first parents, Adam and Eve, and throughout history men's minds have dwelt in the natural darkness which resulted from the fall. "The people who walked in darkness have seen a great light; those who dwelt in a land of deep darkness, on them has light shined" (Isaiah 9:2). That light is Jesus Christ, who has shined in our hearts by the power of the Holy Spirit to bring us out of everlasting night!

But our minds are not renewed overnight. This is plain as Paul addresses the Christians at Rome about their need to resist the pressure of the world and to be "transformed by the renewal of your mind."

"The children of light, being risen with Christ, have a life of their own—the life of pardoned and reconciled believers: renewed in the spirit of their mind, they breathe a new air, they have new interests and affections, and their sympathies are all heavenly and spiritual" *(David Brown: Commentary on Romans 12:2, Critical, Experimental and Practical Commentary, Vol. VI, p. 264).*

As inheritors of the Kingdom of Light, we can choose to live in a continual renewing of our minds, learning more and more to separate light from darkness, good from evil. We *have,* as children of God, the transforming energy of the Holy Spirit to help us in our struggle against our old darkened ways of thinking and to bring us to a new place in Him. No matter where we are in our Christian walk—how new or old, how successful or what failures we have been, we *can* lay hold of that transforming energy by faith through obedience and repentance today. God is with us! Who can be against us!

1. What part does obedience play in the battle for your mind?

2. What part does repentance play in the battle for your mind?

The Mind of Christ

Daily Reading: I Corinthians 2

For who has known the mind of the Lord so as to instruct him? But we have the mind of Christ. (v. 16)

What a startling thing to say! That we actually have available to us with the mind of Christ. C. T. Craig reminds us that Paul is not talking "of the mental faculties with which Jesus was endowed. He means the Spirit which dwelt in Christ, who was himself the Spirit (II Cor. 3:17) and the giver of the Spirit" *(Interpreter's Bible, Vol. 10, p.41).*

This is where the battle for our minds can be won, because Jesus Himself has won the victory over all the powers of hell and darkness, and has given us His Spirit to dwell within every believer. Because of this, we have the light we need, and the help we need, and the thoughts we need, if we will but lay hold on them!

When Paul talks about the spiritual man here in this second chapter of I Corinthians, he is not talking about some few, specially endowed people who are head and shoulders above the rest of us. He is talking about you and me— all who have received Jesus Christ in our hearts by faith. When we receive Him, we receive the Holy Spirit, for God cannot be divided. As He dwells in us, we have access to His light and influence to guide us in our thoughts. It is an exciting, almost unbelievable thing, that God has made His guiding Spirit available to us.

> Holy Spirit, faithful Guide,
> Ever near the Christian's side;
> Gently lead us by the hand,
> Pilgrims in a desert land.
> Weary souls fore'er rejoice
> When they hear that sweetest voice
> Whisper softly, "Wanderer come!
> Follow me, I'll guide thee home."
> *(Marcus M. Wells, 1858)*

We do not struggle alone! God is with us, Christ is for us! Let us never give up!

1. What does it mean to you that you actually have available to you "the mind of Christ"?

2. After this week's emphasis on "Your Mind: A Battleground," what changes have you felt in your daily thought life?

Week Review

All sorts of thoughts invade our minds. We need to do battle against the evil thoughts that invade our minds at the conscious level. As we seek to do battle with our conscious thoughts, the Holy Spirit will do battle for us against any evil thoughts buried at the unconscious level.

1. After the week of study on the mind, and listening to the tape, are you more aware of your thought life? How?

2. Why does this battle seem overwhelming to you?

3. What is your biggest battle in your mind?

SPIRITUAL JOURNAL

It is not safe to have our thought-life dwell on anything but Jesus.

M. Cay & M. Judy

What is Discipleship?

"If any man will come after me, let him deny himself,
and take up his cross daily and follow Me."

Luke 9:23

What Must I Do?

Daily Reading: Mark 10:1-31

And Jesus looking upon him loved him, and said to him, "You lack one thing: go, sell what you have and give to the poor, and you will have treasure in heaven; and come, follow Me, " (v. 21)

One of the most interesting things about this word of Jesus to the rich young man is that He tells him *first* to go and sell what he has and give to the poor, *then* come, follow Me. The first was the means by which he would become a disciple. Discipleship was the goal.

Let's think about that in relation to the past twelve weeks. The diets and disciplines which have been suggested in this 3D program are not ends in themselves. Of course, you wanted to lose (or perhaps to gain) weight. That was a proximate goal which you desired—for good reasons or not-so-good reasons! But the diet and the disciplines were given as the means toward a long-range goal, one harder to reach, yet near at hand: the goal of becoming more genuine followers or disciples of Jesus.

For the rich young man, his money was really not his problem, although it is plain he didn't want to part with it. His real problem was that he did not want to be told what to do! He had rigorously kept "the commandments," meaning that he had built up a tremendous treasure of "rightness," and yet he kept thinking that God required something more. That "something more" was the spontaneous obedience which he would have to display if he was to be a disciple of Jesus Christ. Getting rid of the money was only a first step to free him for such obedience. Getting rid of whatever store of "treasure" we have—self-righteousness, opinions, prejudices, tastes, hurts, resentments,—whatever—is only a way of getting us free to become true disciples, followers, "obedient ones" of Jesus Christ.

How little, then, the price we have paid in these simple disciplines if they lead us toward *this* goal.

A Prayer: *Lord Jesus, I long to be fully and completely Yours. I thank You for the means by which You are setting me free to follow You in whole-hearted obedience. By Your grace, I will follow on. Amen.*

1. How have you learned the blessings of obedience?

Counting the Cost

Daily Reading: Luke 14:15-35

Whoever does not bear his own cross and come after Me, cannot be My disciple. For which of you, desiring to build a tower, does not first sit down and count the cost, whether he has enough to complete it? (vv. 27, 28)

How many projects have you started with good intentions, only to find that after a few days or weeks, the work and struggle grew wearisome, and you gave up? How many diets have you started and did not finish? Or how many resolutions have you made, only to break them before the New Year had scarcely begun?

Counting the cost. What can that mean? Too many people start out their spiritual life with a "gung-ho" attitude, only to find themselves lagging after a few months. It is little wonder that people regard the enthusiasm of a new Christian with some skepticism!

Thomas a Kempis says in his classic devotional book, *The Imitation of Christ:*

Each day we should renew our resolution and bestir ourselves
to fervor, as though it were the first day of our conversion,
and say, "Help me, O Lord, God, in my good resolve and
in your holy service; grant me this day to begin perfectly,
for hitherto I have accomplished nothing."

(Book I, Chapter 19)

Jesus did not quibble about what it was going to cost to be a follower of His. There was no easy, cheap price. He Himself leads the way, by going to the Cross and laying down His own life for our sakes. He warns all who are drawn to Him that there will be a cost involved in finishing our course. Of course it is all grace! We have nothing of ourselves to bring but our need! And what a joy it is that we can begin again, day after day—knowing that His grace is greater than our sins and failures. But we must be prepared to carry through—go all the way. No turning back! That's the key.

A Prayer: *I thank You, Lord Jesus, that You know who I am, and all that I have done, and that You still call me to follow You. No matter what, with Your help, I choose to follow You. Grant me grace to fulfill this good purpose. Amen.*

1. Counting the cost. What does that mean to you?

Let Us Hold True

Daily Reading: Philippians 3

Only let us hold true to what we have attained. (v. 16)

In this chapter, Paul is confessing that he has not yet arrived. "Not that I have already attained this or am already perfect," he says in verse 12. But having confessed this, and his determination to "press on," he admonishes us to hold true to what we have attained.

What have you attained in the twelve weeks of 3D? Have you some weight loss for which you are grateful? Can you see the benefits of the daily disciplines? Are you grateful for the closer sense of fellowship which has grown between members of your group?

Paul knows that not only he, but his readers as well, need to "hold on" to what they have attained in Christ.

The same is true for us. Wherever we are, whatever plateau we may have reached in our upward climb, we need to remember how easy it is to relax, let go, and allow old habit patterns of thought and feeling to dominate us again.

The same temptations which have lured us in wrong paths in the past are all still with us. Our human nature is still vulnerable at certain points to be carried away in hurtful patterns of self-love or self-hate. We still have to fight the feelings of jealousy, the desire to control others, judgmental thoughts, and nursed resentments.

How do we hold true to what we have attained? By remembering who we are, keeping our eyes steadfastly on Jesus and Who He is, and allowing Him free reign to shepherd us through every situation of our lives. By being obedient to the light we have, and being open to more light. By not giving up when the going is tough, and not despairing if we fail!

> I would be true, for there are those who trust me,
> I would be pure, for there are those who care.
> I would be strong, for there is much to suffer,
> I would be brave, for there is much to dare.
>
> *(Howard A. Walter, 1918)*

1. How can you see the benefits of the daily disciplines in your life?

2. How can you keep from letting old habit patterns of thoughts and feelings dominate you again?

Week 12, Day 4

Take My Yoke Upon You

Daily Reading: Matthew 11

Come to Me, all who labor and are heavyladen, and I will give you rest. Take My yoke upon you, and learn from Me; for I am gentle and lowly in heart, and you will find rest for your souls. For My yoke is easy and My burden is light. (vv. 28-30)

As we think about the cost of discipleship, we need also to remember the promise of discipleship. Jesus says that His is an "easy yoke." "Discipleship," says Dietrich Bonhoeffer, "means joy." And he adds, "The command of Jesus is hard, unutterably hard, to those who try to resist it. But for those who willingly submit, the yoke is easy, and the burden is light. 'His commandments are not grievous' (I John 5:3). The commandment of Jesus is not a sort of spiritual shock treatment. Jesus asks nothing of us without giving us the strength to perform it. His commandment never seeks to destroy life, but to foster, strengthen and heal it." *(Cost of Discipleship, pp. 40,41)*

To go on with Jesus from where you are at this moment means coming under His yoke. The oxen is yoked for labor, and is guided by his master. Our yoke is our submission to Jesus, to be guided in all things by Him. He Himself was subject to His Father in all things. The more we subject ourselves to Him, the more complete will be the rest we find for our souls.

"Our hearts are restless till they find their rest in Thee," said St Augustine. He knew that after years of rebellion and looking elsewhere for true satisfaction, that the only rest, true rest, was to be found in subjection to the Lord Jesus Christ.

Discipleship is the continuing path on which we walk as we seek to let our wills become conformed to His will, so that one day, by His grace, we may have the simplicity of heart to have our wills and His be one.

> God doth not need
> Either man's work or his own gifts.
> Who best bear his mild yoke, they serve him best.
> *(John Milton, 1608-1675)*

1. What are you discovering as you submit yourself to Jesus more and more?

His Daily Cross

Daily Reading: Luke 9:7-27

And he said to all, "If any man would come after Me, let him deny himself, and take up his cross daily and follow Me." (v. 23)

What is discipleship? Learning to will what He wills. Learning through pain and failure, through victory and joy that His way is best. Dying daily to the demands of the old nature, allowing oneself to be crossed out without demanding that things go the way one wishes. All this is discipleship.

What is discipleship? To set one's hand to the plow and not turn back. To be one of those who goes on into deeper understanding of God's truth, further repentance for who we are, more absolute dependence on Jesus Christ. All this is discipleship.

What is discipleship? Renewing daily one's love and loyalty to Him who died that we might live. A relationship of Leader and follower. A relationship of growing trust. More of Him and less of me. All this is discipleship.

The Gospel of Luke says it succinctly, that we are to "take up our cross daily" and follow Him. Many are the days when we do not want to take up any cross. We feel we have had enough, and we are tired of fighting against our old Adamic nature. We would rather give in and express the old selves we thought we had left behind!

Beware, disciple! Pray for added grace, and look again at all you have to lose and all you have to gain. Death and sickness, guilt and sin left behind, if we go on with Him. Can we make any other choice!

> Man am I grown, a man's work I must do,
> Follow the dear! follow the Christ, the King,
> Live pure, speak true, right wrong, follow the King—
> Else, wherefore born!

(Alfred Tennyson, 1809-1892)

A Prayer: *Almighty God, whose most dear Son went not up to joy but first He suffered pain, and entered not into glory before He was crucified: mercifully grant that we, walking in the way of the cross may find it none other than the way of life and peace; through the same thy Son Jesus Christ our Lord. Amen.*
(Book of Common Prayer, 1979)

1. What does discipleship mean to you?

I Have Given You an Example

Daily Reading: John 13:1-35

For I have given you an example, that you should do as I have done to you. (v. 15)

In washing the disciples' feet, Jesus, the Lord, took the place of the servant. The act of kneeling down and washing the feet of guests was one of the lowliest of servant-tasks. But this is not just any Rabbi. This is the Lord of Heaven and Earth, stooping to serve fallen mankind.

From the beginning of the Gospels to the very end we have this strange paradox pictured before us—the lowliness of God, the servanthood of Jesus. In His birth, in His life, and in His death there is this strange mixture of lowliness and glory.

What does it mean for us, as far as our discipleship is concerned? He says, "I have given you an example." In the First Letter of Peter, chapter 2, we are told, "For to this you have been called, because Christ also suffered for you, leaving you an example that you should follow in His steps" (v. 21). We are to look to His life as our pattern, not just as a means of our salvation from sin. He has lived as we are called to live.

In another place He says, "I came not to do my own will, but the will of Him who sent me." That is an example for us.

And again He says, "My food is to do the will of Him who sent me and to finish His work." That is an example.

In the garden of Gethsemane, He said, "Father, if it is possible, let this cup pass from Me. Nevertheless, not what I will, but Thy will be done." That is an example for us.

As we look and learn from Him, let us pray that His image will be formed in us, His life grow in us, so that what we shall be, will be like Him.

> O to be like Thee! Blessed Redeemer,
> This is my constant longing and prayer.
> Gladly I'll forfeit all of earth's treasures,
> Jesus, Thy perfect likeness to wear.
> O to be like Thee, Blessed Redeemer,
> Pure as Thou art;
> Come in Thy sweetness, come in Thy fullness;
> Stamp Thine own image deep on my heart.
> *(Thomas O. Chisholm)*

1. The "lowliness of God"—What does that mean to you in your daily life?

If Anyone Serves Me

Daily Reading: John 12:20-50

If any one serve Me, he must follow Me; and where I am, there shall My servant be also; if any one serves Me, the Father will honor him. (v. 26)

We have come to the end of our twelve weeks of the first session of 3D. It has, no doubt, been a mixture of joy and pain, success and failure, fun and work. But in it all, we have been walking with Jesus Christ our Lord. Our aim has been to learn better how to serve and follow Him.

Now we must go on with our lives—either in further sessions of 3D or in our other forms of commitment to Him. In any case, here is both a warning and a promise in today's verse.

First, the warning. If we are to serve Jesus, we must follow Him. It is not a matter of "being good," "doing the right thing," obeying the Law, or doing good works. It is a matter of following the Living Christ. He is alive, He has a will for us, and He is present with us. Let that reality become more and more a part of your daily consciousness. Brother Lawrence was a cook in a French monastery in the 17th century. He learned a wonderful secret, since retold many times in a little book called *The Practice of the Presence of God.* He says,

> I make it my only business to persevere in His holy Presence, wherein I keep myself by a simple attention and an absorbing passionate regard to God, which I may call an *actual presence of God*; or, to speak better, a silent and secret conversation of the soul with God . . . .

Second, the promise. Jesus says, "If any one serves Me, the Father will honor him." That is His promise, and you can depend on it. No one truly serves and loves the Son who is not honored by the Father Himself. What greater reward could we ask, what great enticement to the way of discipleship?

> If I find Him, if I follow
> Is He sure to bless?
> Saints, apostles, prophets, martyrs
> Answer, "Yes!"

A Prayer: *Thank You, Father, for the disciplines and the joys of these past weeks. Thank You for beginning a new work of grace and love in my life. Bless all who traveled with me, and grant us grace to go on, knowing that the way leads home. In Jesus' Name. Amen.*

1. What have these weeks of discipline meant to you?

Week Review

We are so pleased you have completed these twelve weeks. We know you have been blessed, and that you have had success with your diet. Now that you've been part of a 3D experience, you can now be aware that there are definite areas in your life where you need God's help.

1. What are these areas of need?

2. What weekly Bible Study and Daily Devotional subject was most helpful to you? Why?

3. What is the ultimate goal of your life?

We pray that you will continue on in 3D, and allow the work which God has begun through the 3D program to be completed in you.

We pray God's richest blessing upon you.

SPIRITUAL JOURNAL

We must allow the work that Christ has done in us to be established in us.

M. Cay & M. Judy

Congratulations!

When you joined the 3D program you expected to lose some weight. You were presented with an excellent food plan, good nutritional information and a challenge to exercise. Most importantly, you had a desire to participate in a support group program and to learn to bring your whole life under the direction of God.

We pray that you have seen some fruit from these twelve weeks. The truth is, it will take most of us a lot longer than twelve weeks to change our eating habits and our opinions related to food and exercise or discipline. Many of us are undisciplined, but it is never too late to change. You have started to walk in the right direction, and we are glad if the 3D program has been instrumental in teaching you about basic Christian truths. While you may have lost weight, we know you have gained—spiritually! And that is what 3D is all about.

Now we want to challenge you further—towards growth and maturity in Christ within the 3D program. The next devotional workbook is called The Heart of the Matter. The daily readings provided walk you through many of life's struggles in a down to earth, honest and realistic way. Through Bible reading, sharing, and your support group, you will begin to recognize roadblocks in your life that affect everything from the way you eat to the way you relate to other people and, most importantly, the way you relate to God. This devotional will encourage and motivate you in your daily walk.

Be sure to take notice of the additional materials available through 3D. If you want information about low fat eating and strength training exercises, inquire about the Free From Fat program. If you are interested in other devotional workbooks, ask for Pressing On and Along the King's Highway. We have many other books and videos available as well. The Taste of New Wine by Keith Miller and Fruit from the Vine by Alice Flaherty are two excellent titles, both dealing with everyday Christian living.

Be faithful and expect great things from God!

Commit Yourself to a New Start

3D introduces
Action Kit II
36 weeks of life-changing devotionals

Heart of the Matter
Pressing On
Along the King's Highway

For the first time, 3D is offering **Action Kit II** to encourage you to
continue in the 3D program. On its own, Action Kit II is an inspirational
set for anyone looking for practical answers to real-life problems.
Whether you are in a 3D group or not, these devotionals will spur you
on in the Christian life. **$32.95**

Action Kit II Teaching Tapes are now available to supplement the
devotionals. These six cassettes can offer additional short teachings for
each week. Excellent for further personal meditation or group
discussion. **$33.95**

Up With Weights and Down With Fats

Free From Fat

3D presents **Free From Fat**, a program that will put down the drudgery, discontent and disappointment of every dieter! Instead you will find encouragement and new enthusiasm while learning basic new insights on low fat eating and strength training exercise. Not only will you learn the facts, but without a lot of effort you will be able to apply them to your daily life.

This set includes a guide and a 263 page cookbook from the Henry Ford Heart and Vascular Institute called *Heart Smart*. It provides complete nutritional information, including food exchanges, cholesterol, and grams of fat.

Free From Fat Kit   **$21.95**

FREE SHIPPING WITH THIS COUPON

ORDER TODAY!

Send this coupon to:
3D, P.O. Box 897, Orleans, MA 02653

or call the 3D office at:
1-800-451-5006 and be sure to mention this free shipping offer!

Free From Fat Kit

Please send me _____ sets of the Free From Fat program at $21.95 per set.

☐ Check   ☐ Charge

Acct # _____ Exp. _____

Name _____

Address_____

City/State/Zip _____

Phone # _____

WB1-2

How to cope with life—and win!

Fruit from the Vine

What do you do when you're hurting so badly, you don't feel like praying? When you have difficulty thinking of God as a loving Father? When it seems as if He is indifferent to your plight or your suffering? Ever feel discouraged? Read this book.

Sometimes it's hard to imagine spiritual giants of our era having crises of faith . . . but they do, and some have had the courage and honesty to share them. As we see them facing the same sturggles that we do, we can take heart: like them, we, too, can come through this trial stronger. For the Lord prunes His vines that they might bring forth good fruit . . . and some of the best from Catherine Marshall, Joni Eareckson, Bruce Larsen, Colleen Townsend Evans, Peter Kreeft, Terry Fullam, and others can be found in this book. **$8.95**

FREE SHIPPING WITH THIS COUPON

ORDER TODAY!

Send this coupon to:
3D, P.O. Box 897, Orleans, MA 02653

or call the 3D office at:
1-800-451-5006 and be sure to mention this free shipping offer!

Fruit from the Vine

Please send me _____ copies of Fruit from the Vine at $8.95 each.

☐ Check ☐ Charge

Acct # _____ Exp. _____

Name _____

Address_____

City/State/Zip _____

Phone # _____

WB1-3

3D *Food Sheet* _____ Name _____

Daily Calories _____ Week: _____

Food Exchanges	Day 1	2	3	4	5	6	7	
BREAKFAST Meat								
Bread								
Fruit								
Milk								
Fat								
LUNCH Meat								
Bread								
Vegetable								
Fruit								
Milk								
Fat								
DINNER Meat								
Bread								
Vegetable								
Fruit								
Milk								
Fat								
EXTRA:								

3D *Food Sheet* Name _____ Daily Calories _____ Week: _____

Food Exchanges		Day 1		2		3		4		5		6		7	
BREAKFAST	Meat														
	Bread														
	Fruit														
	Milk														
	Fat														
LUNCH	Meat														
	Bread														
	Vegetable														
	Fruit														
	Milk														
	Fat														
DINNER	Meat														
	Bread														
	Vegetable														
	Fruit														
	Milk														
	Fat														
EXTRA:															

3D Food Sheet

Name: _____ Daily Calories _____ Week: _____

Food Exchanges	Day 1	2	3	4	5	6	7
BREAKFAST Meat							
Bread							
Fruit							
Milk							
Fat							
LUNCH Meat							
Bread							
Vegetable							
Fruit							
Milk							
Fat							
DINNER Meat							
Bread							
Vegetable							
Fruit							
Milk							
Fat							
EXTRA:							

3D *Food Sheet* Name _____ Daily Calories _____ Week: _____

Food Exchanges		Day 1		2		3		4		5		6		7	
BREAKFAST	Meat														
	Bread														
	Fruit														
	Milk														
	Fat														
LUNCH	Meat														
	Bread														
	Vegetable														
	Fruit														
	Milk														
	Fat														
DINNER	Meat														
	Bread														
	Vegetable														
	Fruit														
	Milk														
	Fat														
EXTRA:															

3D *Food Sheet* Name _____ Daily Calories _____ Week: _____

Food Exchanges	Day 1	2	3	4	5	6	7
BREAKFAST Meat							
Bread							
Fruit							
Milk							
Fat							
LUNCH Meat							
Bread							
Vegetable							
Fruit							
Milk							
Fat							
DINNER Meat							
Bread							
Vegetable							
Fruit							
Milk							
Fat							
EXTRA:							

3D *Food Sheet*   Name _____   Daily Calories _____   Week: _____

Food Exchanges	Day 1	2	3	4	5	6	7	
BREAKFAST Meat / Bread / Fruit / Milk / Fat								
LUNCH Meat / Bread / Vegetable / Fruit / Milk / Fat								
DINNER Meat / Bread / Vegetable / Fruit / Milk / Fat								
EXTRA:								

COMMITMENT CARD

Name _____

Address _____

City/State/Zip _____

Telephone _____

Church _____

Age _____ Present Weight _____ Goal Weight _____

How long have you been overweight? _____

How long have you been underweight? _____

Are you under a doctor's care? _____

Do you exercise? _____ Do you take vitamins? _____

Why do you want to join 3D? _____

_____

Continued on Reverse Side

3D *Diet, Discipline and Discipleship*

COMMITMENT PRAYER

I ask for God's strength to operate through me as I commit myself to:

1. Attend 3D meetings

2. Maintain Daily Devotions

3. To care and pray daily for the other members in my group

4. Memorize Weekly Scripture Verse

5. Exercise regularly

6. Share openly and honestly with my 3D support group

_____

Signature   Date